Positional Release Technique

Positional Release Technique
From a Dynamic Systems Perspective

Denise Deig, M.S.P.T., G.C.F.P.

Clinic Director, Broad Ripple, Physiotherapy Associates, Indianapolis

Forewords by

Carol A. Montgomery, M.S., P.T.

*Physical Therapist, Integrated Medicine Center and Rehabilitation Center,
Columbus Regional Hospital, Columbus, Indiana*

and

Amy D. Konkle, M.D.

*Clinical Associate Professor of Psychiatry, Indiana University School of Medicine, Indianapolis;
Psychiatrist, St. Vincent Stress Centers, Indianapolis*

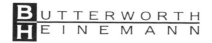

BUTTERWORTH
HEINEMANN

Boston Oxford Auckland Johannesburg Melbourne New Delhi

Every effort has been made to ensure that the drug dosage schedules within this text are accurate and conform to standards accepted at time of publication. However, as treatment recommendations vary in the light of continuing research and clinical experience, the reader is advised to verify drug dosage schedules herein with information found on product information sheets. This is especially true in cases of new or infrequently used drugs.

 Recognizing the importance of preserving what has been written, Butterworth–Heinemann prints its books on acid-free paper whenever possible.

 Butterworth–Heinemann supports the efforts of American Forests and the Global ReLeaf program in its campaign for the betterment of trees, forests, and our environment.

Library of Congress Cataloging-in-Publication Data

Deig, Denise.
    Positional release technique : from a dynamic systems perspective / Denise Deig.
      p. cm.
    Includes bibliographical references and index.
    ISBN 0-7506-7225-0
    1. Manipulation (Therapeutics) I. Title.

RM724 .D45 2000
615.8'2—dc21

            00-026041

British Library Cataloguing-in-Publication Data
A catalogue record for this book is available from the British Library.

The publisher offers special discounts on bulk orders of this book.
For information, please contact:

Manager of Special Sales
Butterworth–Heinemann
225 Wildwood Avenue
Woburn, MA 01801-2041
Tel: 781-904-2500
Fax: 781-904-2620

For information on all Butterworth–Heinemann publications available, contact our World Wide Web home page at: http://www.bh.com

10 9 8 7 6 5 4 3 2 1

Printed in the United States of America

Contents

Foreword

Denise Deig is commended for her creative and detailed presentation of a complex and controversial paradigm shift that is taking place within evaluation and treatment strategies, as well as in patient-therapist relationships within the field of physical therapy. In the last five years, interest in the manual approach to evaluation and treatment has surged. This is evidenced by the plethora of continuing education courses offered regarding manual therapy procedures, the significant increase in curricular time allotted to manual therapy techniques within entry-level physical therapy education programs, and the acute rise in the number of consumers seeking treatment from private practice body workers.

Likewise, a parallel interest in the effects of manual therapies can be observed within the medical community, as demonstrated by presentations at annual meetings in the fields of neurology, psychology, and psychiatry. Even the federal government has acknowledged the sweeping rise and effectiveness of manual therapy by making recent changes in their publications of the current procedural terminology (CPT) and reimbursement codes.

Despite this wide interest and publicity, there continues to be a deficit in the scientific literature regarding the role of the nervous system in the efficacy of some forms of manual therapy. Chapter 2, "Theoretical Foundations," begins a stimulating discussion and demonstrates Deig's laborious efforts to provide a comprehensive framework for the reasons why indirect techniques, including Positional Release, work. Additionally, the thorough literature review of the various disciplines underlines the importance of a multifaceted approach in evaluating and treating each individual as an integrated human being rather than as a diagnosis or a "one-system dysfunction."

Given my extensive studies of body-mind theory, what excites me about *Positional Release Technique* is Deig's ability to offer language that promotes discussion and thought regarding multiple systems that effect healing. Where most authors have focused on one or two areas, Deig's book is metaphorically like the "nervous system" itself. She discusses the widespread influence of "interneuronal connections" to other "systems," such as sociology, psychology, mathematics, and physics. Deig offers the reader a possible bridge that explains how the synaptic cleft between physical intervention and emotional release is very small indeed. Although targeted for the professional audience of physical and occupational therapists, Deig's *Positional Release Technique* would also be of interest to other somatic body workers, including massage therapists, chiropractors, physicians, and individuals working in the field of psychology.

In writing *Positional Release Technique*, Deig displays significant courage in broaching a subject that can be controversial and largely supported by anecdotal literature. Interestingly, one of the great benefits of this book is her careful and precise construction of a manual that standardizes Positional Release technique. This will enable others to study Positional Release technique through outcomes and efficacy research in the future. As professionals and clinicians, we have a responsibility to our patients and our profession to apply techniques that work. Deig's book challenges us to look at our own clinical results and outcomes as we apply these techniques.

Deig is a talented clinician, an innovative pioneer, and a model for the other clinical physical therapists. She demonstrates that it is possible to practice as a full-time clinician, teach entry-level and postprofessional students, and contribute to the field of research.

Carol A. Montgomery, M.S., P.T.

Foreword

The past 15 years have seen the rise of a renewed focus on the understanding and treatment of trauma. Neurochemical and neuroimaging research has told us much about the neurophysiology and functional neuroanatomy of trauma; clinical observation and research tells us how far we still have to go in being able to reverse its effects. The author brings the physical therapist a step closer toward that goal.

Trauma is rampant in our society. It ranges on a continuum of causes and severity, and rarely, if ever, does trauma exist purely as physical or psychological in nature. Many in the psychological trauma field, including leading clinical researchers, emphasize the necessity of dealing with the body when trying to facilitate healing from trauma of the sort previously thought of as psychological in nature. Schools of body-oriented psychotherapy have evolved, such as Hakomi and Somatic Experiencing techniques. Eye movement desensitization and reprocessing (EMDR), one of the most empirically validated treatments for posttraumatic stress disorder, includes somatic sensation in its protocol for processing, regardless of the nature of the trauma. And, regardless of the nature of the trauma, EMDR patients who are accessing the memory of a trauma by calling up a visual image (or memory of sound, smell, taste, or touch), cognition and affect are usually able to identify somatosensory elements, although they may not previously have connected the somatosensory cues to the trauma.

It is important to note that the experience of any one element of the traumatic memory trace may evoke the experience of some of all of the other elements. Hence, the process of physical therapy, by recreating somatosensory phenomena related to the traumatic experience, may trigger visual images, emotions, and self-perceptions also related to the trauma. Because memory of traumatic experience tends to be stored in fragmented form rather than as a cohesive unit, the patient may not know why he or she is reacting in such a manner.

As the methods for facilitating the healing of psychological trauma have begun to improve, so has there been an increase in awareness of the continuum of trauma and the effect of smaller traumas; that is, traumas not ordinarily perceived as catastrophic on the day-to-day functioning of humans and their emotional and physical well-being. These traumas may include falls, serious illness, even apparently minor automobile accidents, medical procedures, and surgeries, to mention only a few. The experience of prior traumatization, whether of an apparently similar nature or not, may complicate the response to and healing from current trauma.

The ways in which other emotional factors potentially influence a course of physical therapy and response to therapy are myriad. Anxiety or depression may exist secondary to the presenting symptom cluster or to its causative trauma or disorder, or it may be present coincidentally. Either or both may affect both the quality and the intensity of pain. The ability of the patient to carry out exercises at home may be impaired by difficulties in attention, memory, energy, interest, and motivation. Nutrition may be poor due to appetite changes or lack of energy or motivation to prepare food. Adequate sleep and rest for healing may be impaired. Anxiety may increase muscle tension and spasm and slow the return to normal muscle position and function. Apparent overreaction to stimuli, if not accurately perceived and attended to by the therapist, may set up tension and misunderstanding between patient and therapist, and undermine the effective communication and cooperation, impeding the process of recovery. Conscious or unconscious secondary gain may further influence the treatment course.

Deig offers her readers a broad view of ongoing patient assessment that includes attention to emotional and psychological factors and offers practical ways to incorporate that assessment into treatment. Our patients are not well served by strict compartmentalization by their providers of medical care. The best care takes into account the whole of the person, even though the primary focus is on the area of the provider's expertise.

I know from personal experience the wide range of technical knowledge and expertise, the skill, the compassion, and the gentle effectiveness that Denise Deig brings to her work as a physical therapist. Her students should consider themselves fortunate to have her as a teacher and a role model. I applaud her integrative approach and dedication to the inclusion of the whole human system in her attentiveness, perception, and treatment approach. Ideally, her stance is part of a leading edge within our broader health care delivery system.

Amy D. Konkle, M.D.

Preface

My purpose in writing this book is to introduce practitioners to an indirect treatment approach that is easy to learn and will provide a nonforceful alternative for patient care. My unique method of treatment is friendly to both therapist and patient alike. This is accomplished by applying osteopathic-based theoretical concepts to a physical therapy frame of reference, using applied anatomy and joint mobilization skills. The emphasis is not on memorizing specific tender points and release positions but on using and expanding on an existing skill and knowledge base of anatomy, joint mobilization, and evaluation tools. Therefore, the focus is on understanding the underlying philosophy and the reason for application of the treatment techniques described, as well as development of observation, palpation, and patient-handling skills by the therapist.

My initial exposure to indirect techniques was through Arthur Pauls, a British osteopath who developed Ortho-Bionomy®. After several years of study, I became an Ortho-Bionomy instructor and, in 1982, began teaching this method. I found these studies very formative in developing the Positional Release technique described in this book. However, when I taught Ortho-Bionomy to physical therapists, they found the work interesting and useful but also frustrating to learn and apply, due to the lack of structure and the esoteric nature of the method. The physical therapy frame of reference used in this book may lend clarity to this material and facilitate the learning process for practitioners.

My study of indirect osteopathic work includes several classes on Strain-CounterStrain® taught through the Jones Institute. I have also had the privilege of studying Functional Method with Ed Stiles, D.O., whose comprehensive understanding and insights substantially contribute to the ongoing development of indirect work. Elements of all the indirect techniques I have studied are blended and developed into a physical therapy framework, resulting in the Positional Release technique presented in this publication.

Dynamic Systems Theory (DST) serves as an important and integral foundation for the context of this book for several reasons. First, it allows me to describe most clearly the clinical experience I have gathered in my 25 years of physical therapy practice. It also allows me to develop a model for evaluation, intervention, and the patient-therapist relationship that is consistent with the underlying osteopathic philosophy, the techniques presented, and my worldview.

My formal introduction to DST was in a Theoretical Foundations for Evaluation and Treatment of Neurologic Dysfunctions course offered at the University of Indianapolis, while attaining my masters degree. Prior to this, I was exposed to systems concepts by in-depth discussions with two friends, both professors in different fields. One is a theologian, Ursula Pflafflin, who teaches theology and psychology with a family systems focus. The other is a chemistry professor, Raima Larter, who is well versed in chaos theory and currently is writing a textbook on the subject. More recently, the Feldenkrais® community has begun to relate and discuss systems theory with regard to their work.

From a systems perspective, there is a new sense of awareness of the importance of honoring and respecting the uniqueness of each individual. The patient's subjective experience and emergent response to therapeutic intervention becomes significant, as does the therapist's observations. Evaluation becomes more than collection of objective data. A dynamic circular process of continuous reevaluation evolves and guides the treatment process and direction. My goal in writing this book is to create a bridge for traditionally trained therapists to make the transition into a more holistic systems approach to evaluation, treatment, and patient-therapist relationships.

At the heart of developing a new type of relationship between therapist and patient lies the issue of force. For too long, popular sayings associated discomfort with physical therapy treatment; these include "no pain, no gain," and our initials (PT) with "pain and torture" or "physical torture." I believe that our profession is at a point of evolution where we are now ready to move away from these combative representations of the patient-therapist relationship into a model based on gentle intervention and enhanced awareness. If we can accomplish the same or greater goals and patient outcomes using gentler methods such as the one presented in this book, why would we choose to do otherwise?

In my practice, I continuously blend direct and indirect techniques, based on patient diagnosis and response. When shifting into a direct approach I attempt to take the same measure of sensitivity and awareness that I developed in my indirect focus. This assures me of not engaging in a tug of war with the patient's tissues and minimizes or eliminates treatment trauma. Please think about how much trauma the patient's system may have sustained by the time physical therapy treatment is initiated and as you consider intervention options. The techniques presented here allow therapists to have a treatment model based on gentler and more aware intervention at their disposal.

Medicine at large is changing in ways that are consistent with this new systems understanding and awareness. Recent statistics on the numbers of people who seek alternative care shocked many physicians and other health care professionals.[1,2] This has prompted an emergence of integrative heath centers across the United States in the past several years. While we have gathered a wealth of information in specialty medicine, we may be at a crossroad where it is time to reunite the parts and find ways to treat the patient as a whole.

As we begin to treat the whole person, it is imperative that we bring an increased awareness of the impact our interventions may have into our scope of practice. For example, the issue of underlying emotional considerations during physical therapy treatment recently has been described in a revealing qualitative study in our professional journal.[3] In this study, survivors of childhood sexual abuse described their response to physical therapy interventions and gave suggestions for more sensitive handling during therapy. Sensitive practice included providing a sense of safety during treatment, consideration of the client's emotional history and well-being, increasing awareness of emotional triggers during physical interventions, establishing a sense of relationship with the client, and practicing in a holistic fashion. My clinical experience echoes the findings of this study, as the impact of a quiet touch often evokes patient insights and emotional expressions beyond any imagining. The practice of Positional Release technique as described in this book may provide further insight into issues of sensitivity and awareness in physical therapy practice.

My undergraduate degree in Psychology and both formal and informal postgraduate study in this field have increased my comfort level in handling occurrences of emotional response during physical therapy. I also have developed a very positive working relationship with several psychotherapists and the psychiatrist Amy Konkle, who wrote a Foreword to this book. When given permission, I do not hesitate to consult with a patient's psychological counselor or make referrals as necessary. Many of the patients seeking physical therapy intervention require an increased sensitivity and a cross-disciplinary approach to care. I think it is both possible and necessary to sensibly address the cross-discipline issues of body-mind and somatoemotional responses by complementing rather than compromising our individual scopes of professional practice.

I also would like to mention that I am a guild-certified Feldenkrais practitioner (GCFP). This training process and its clinical applications have been influential in my physical therapy practice. Although this book will not cover the Feldenkrais method in any depth, the influence is pervasive. Therefore, Dynamic Systems Theory and the Feldenkrais method, which are quite consistent with each other as well as with Positional Release technique as presented, provide the underlying tone and perspective for this book.

The obvious lack of outcome studies on the techniques presented here and indirect methods in general may be cited as a weakness for this method and publication. The need for further research studies on indirect methods is clear. For this book, the eight case studies[4] in Part III and the one unpublished research study by Annis in Chapter 2 will have to be considered as the current outcome measures available. I hope that the clinical observations presented here will spark enough interest in indirect work to encourage further investigation.

Positional Release techniques, as presented in this book, have a broad clinical application. Although the book is written primarily for the physical therapist, a number of other health care professionals could benefit from learning this method. Occupational therapists, athletic trainers, doctors, nurses, Feldenkrais practitioners, and massage therapists are among the practitioners who may have the interest and skill base to learn some or all of this material.

The book is organized into three parts. The first part is an introduction to indirect osteopathic and dynamic systems theory principles and theoretical foundation. This includes a historical and comparative review of other indirect methods. Examination, evaluation, treatment intervention, and patient response also are discussed.

The second part of this book was originally developed as a teaching manual for Positional Release courses, which I taught for more than 15 years. This part includes muscular and joint applications as well as isometric exercises. A thorough knowledge of anatomy is an important prerequisite to learning the muscular application techniques. The anatomical drawings here should be useful in facilitating this learning process. In fact, I recommend that therapy students would benefit from the anatomical review and application in this section.

Some joint mobilization skills are necessary to learn the joint application techniques. However, application can be made to any mobilization skills in which the reader is versed, not just the techniques described in the book. The isometrics chapter is only a brief glimpse into the possibilities available, as I would suggest that nearly all the releases described could include an isometric component. However, I have omitted extensive descriptions due to space considerations.

The final part of the book is devoted to case studies of eight clinical applications of Positional Release technique. These case studies have been gathered from students during 10 years of teaching a Positional Release courses in postprofessional graduate programs at the University of Indianapolis. A case study involving Positional Release technique was the postcourse requirement for students who enrolled in the three-credit-hour course. I have chosen seven representative case studies to highlight a wide scope of clinical application and the integration with other treatment methods. In these case studies, students were not required to use Positional Release in isolation, which is consistent with my view of the role it holds in physical therapy practice. The final case study is from my current clinical practice.

Finally, I invite you to be creative in applying the techniques discussed here in your own practice. The releases, as described, are guidelines based on anatomical and other scientific and therapeutic knowledge. They are not prescriptive in nature, nor do they represent a final evolution of the concepts. One of my greatest fears in writing this book is that placing this information in a published form would limit the possibilities to only those described. However, discussing systems theory in relationship to the ideas presented here brings the work alive for me, and my hope is that this enthusiasm will come through the pages to your hands.

Denise Deig, M.S.P.T., G.C.F.P.

References

1. Eisenberg DM, Kessler RC, Foster C, et al. Unconventional medicine in the United States. *NEGL J Med.* 1993;328:246–252.
2. Eisenberg DM, Davis RB, Ettner SL, et al. Trends in alternative medicine use in the United States 1990–1997: Results of a follow-up national survey. *JAMA* November 1998;280: 1569–1575.
3. Schachter CL, Stalker CA, Teram E. Toward sensitive practice: Issues for physical therapists working with survivors of childhood sexual abuse. *Phys Ther.* 1999;79:248–261.
4. Lukoff D, Edwards D, Miller M. The case study as a scientific method for researching alternative therapies. *Alternative Therapies.* 1993;4:44–52.

Acknowledgments

I would like to thank Kim Watanabe, physical therapist and artist, for her significant contribution as illustrator of this book. The 63 original anatomical line and figure drawings and the cover artwork are representative of her wide-ranging artistic talents. Kim worked unselfishly on this project against demanding time constraints and deadlines. She consistently and cheerfully met these demands in spite of personal health concerns that would have deterred anyone with less dedication and commitment. In addition, she gave me considerable support and encouragement during the writing and editorial process as well as offering her valuable insight regarding the written material.

I also acknowledge Connie McCloy, Ed.D., P.T., A.T.C., director of the DPT Program at the University of Indianapolis, for her unselfish contribution to this book. Her editorial suggestions, research assistance, and support were considerable during an extensive revision phase. Her critical eye and efforts led to a final manuscript consistent with physical therapy professional standards with a stronger theoretical research foundation.

Patricia Proffitt, M.S., P.T., my longtime business partner and Positional Release teaching assistant, and Carol Montgomery, M.S., P.T., also were instrumental in reviewing this manuscript. Patricia assisted with sections on Positional Release technique, manual therapy, and references to the Jones Strain-CounterStrain® method. Carol lent her expertise in the areas of manual therapy, the Feldenkrais® method, and body-mind integration, with her background in Gestalt and other psychotherapeutic processes. Two additional physical therapists, Mary Delaney, M.S., P.T., owner of Innovative Therapy Services, and Sam Kegerreis, M.S., P.T., A.T.C., professor at the University of Indianapolis, reviewed the manuscript in its early phase and offered their valuable insight and feedback.

Manuscript reviewers with expertise outside the field of physical therapy include: Raima Larter, Ph.D., chemistry professor at Indiana University–Purdue University Indianapolis (IUPUI); Amy Konkle, M.D., psychiatrist at St. Vincent Stress Centers and clinical associate professor of Psychiatry at Indiana University School of Medicine; Elizabeth Gaines, M.S. (Vocational Rehabilitation), M.A., L.C.S.W. (Ph.D. candidate); and LuAnn Overmyer, B.A., advanced Ortho-Bionomy® instructor. Raima assisted with extensive consulting and editing on the physics and nonlinear dynamics portion of the book. Amy and Elizabeth provided very valuable insights from the fields of psychiatry, psychology, social work, and vocational rehabilitation. LuAnn lent steadfast enthusiasm and support to this project as well as providing specifics regarding the practice of Ortho-Bionomy.

Finally, I would like to acknowledge the seven University of Indianapolis postprofessional students whose case studies appear in Part III of this book. These written contributions were made by Michelle Jones, Wendel Lamason, Tricia Mahoney, Heidi E. Baumeister, Stacey M. Reeves, Andrea Phillips, and Lynne Patterson. I appreciate the clinical insights and observations of these physical therapists as well as their cooperation with the editorial process.

I am grateful to every one of these dedicated professionals for their assistance with this project. I am honored to have these remarkable health care providers, teachers, and friends as part of my own system of support. Without the friendship, honesty, and assistance of these colleagues, this book would not have been possible.

Positional Release Technique

Part I

Conceptual Model and Methodology

1

Introduction to Indirect Methods and Dynamic Systems Theory

Origins of Direct and Indirect Techniques

The terminology of direct and indirect techniques originated in the field of osteopathy. In the 1940s, Hoover[1] classified direct and indirect techniques as follows:

> *(1) Direct technique: the method of moving one bone or segment of the articular lesion directly to a normal relationship with its neighbor. This is accomplished against the resistance of tissues and fluids maintaining the abnormal relationship . . . (2) Indirect technic: the method of moving one bone or segment slightly in the direction away from the direction of correction until the resistance of holding tissues and fluids is partially overcome and the tensions are bilaterally balanced; then allowing the released ligaments and muscles themselves to aid in pulling the part toward normal.*

In *Principles of Manual Medicine,*[2] Greenman defined direct procedures as those that directly engage the restrictive joint barrier or resistant soft tissues. He stated that, although high-velocity, low-amplitude thrusting procedures are most usually direct, they also have been described as an indirect procedure termed rebound thrust. He classified myofascial release and craniosacral techniques as either direct or indirect and related that they sometimes are used in combination. Functional technique and Strain-CounterStrain® consistently are designated indirect techniques in the literature.

For the purposes of this book, the following definition of *direct* and *indirect techniques* are used: Direct joint techniques include those that go against the restrictive barrier, while indirect joint techniques include those that go away from the restrictive barrier. When considering the soft tissue releases, direct techniques include those that involve stretching muscles or going into tissue restriction, while indirect techniques include those that involve shortening muscles or going away from tissue restriction.

Classification of Direct and Indirect Techniques

Tables 1-1 and 1-2 may help clarify how many current methods typically are classified as direct or indirect. Please note the exceptions referred to previously by Greenman. Muscle energy techniques, for example, almost always are described as direct but also can be done indirectly, depending on patient response and other considerations.

Table 1-1 Joint Techniques

Direct	Indirect
Manipulation	Functional technique[3]
Mobilization	Strain-CounterStrain[4]
High-velocity, low-amplitude direct thrust	Positional Release joint application
Muscle energy[2]	(Muscle energy)
(Craniosacral)[5]	Craniosacral

Note: When a technique appears in parentheses it is thought to be used in that category less often.

Table 1-2 Myofascial Techniques

Direct	Indirect
Cross friction and cross fiber—Pfrimmer[6]	Positional Release muscular application
Deep soft tissue work	Positional Release isometrics
Postural integration—Rolfing[7]	Functional integration—Feldenkrais*[8]
Myofascial stretching	Myofascial shortening

*The Feldenkrais method is defined as somatic education. Functional integration sessions involve dynamic movement and postural work focused on specific functions, with occasional handling similar to indirect methods.

Osteopathic Origins

Since Positional Release technique is consistent with the osteopathic philosophy established by Still in the 1800s, it is briefly reviewed here. Andrew Taylor Still, the founder of osteopathy, was trained as a medical doctor but was disenchanted by the practice of medicine in his day.[2,9] His philosophy of medicine, which helps define the fundamental concepts in the osteopathic field to this day, includes the following:

- Unity of the body.
- Healing power of nature.
- Role of physician was to enhance the body's ability to heal and recover from disease.
- Somatic component of disease.
- Structure-function interrelationship.
- Total body integration.
- Benefits of manipulative therapy in restoring maximum function and wellness.
- Innate intelligence of brain and central nervous system.

These concepts clearly establish Still as an early proponent of the integrative principles found in dynamic systems theory and are entirely consistent with the Positional Release principles presented here.

Current osteopathic writings echo much of Still's earlier work, supporting the role of manual therapy in medicine. Greenman viewed the musculoskeletal system from a broad and integrative perspective that is related to the total organism and stated five basic concepts, which are interrelated and influence all functional aspects.[2] These five concepts are holistic (treat the host, not the disease), neurological, circulatory, energy-spending (musculoskeletal), and self-regulating man.

Dynamic Systems Theory

The concepts of Dynamic Systems Theory (DST) have begun to influence thinking in a wide range of physical and behavioral sciences. In the field of physical therapy, systems theory is more familiar to clinicians specializing in neurology than those trained in orthopedics. For example, DST has been researched extensively in the field of child development and motor learning. Esther Thelen,[10,11] a psychologist at Indiana University, led the way in this research and what has evolved is an entirely new perspective on how a child's movement patterns and cognition develop. She stated,

What the motor studies have shown us, however, is that each component in the developing system is both cause and product [and] . . . From a dynamic point of view, therefore, the developmental questions are not what abilities or core knowledge infants and children really "have" or what parts of their behavior are truly organic or genetic but how the parts cooperate to produce stability or engender change.[10]

She further discussed the genetics verses environment and structure verses function debates and concluded that causality is not even the issue:

> *Rather, the new synthesis sees everything as a dynamic process, albeit on different levels and time scales. Even what psychologists usually call "structure"—the tissues and organs of the body—is a dynamic process. Bones and muscles are continually in flux, although their changes may be slower and less observable than those in the nervous system.*[10]

And finally, regarding intervention, she stated, "Instead, the therapist needs to know the history of the system in all its richness and complexity, its current dynamics, and how the interventions can disrupt the stability of the current dynamics to allow new and better solutions to emerge."[10]

These eloquent quotes are pertinent to the field of physical therapy at large. Radical shifts in thinking are evolving in our field and in science as a whole, most refer to this as a paradigm shift. Inherent in this paradigm shift are new discoveries in the field of physics—often referred to as *new physics, quantum physics,* and *chaos theory.*[12–15] Table 1-3 is a comparative summary of a more traditionally oriented perspective to a dynamic systems perspective, with a focus on the issues and concepts most pertinent to physical therapy.

Table 1-3 does not reflect right or wrong perspectives, rather, it is an expansion of how we potentially can relate to patient care. There are many evaluation tools, tests, and standards of practice that define our profession and indeed benefit our patients. However, there are times when professional tools can limit rather than facilitate our understanding of what is going on with a patient. In many areas, we could improve and expand our patient-therapist relationship and begin to treat patients in a more integrated fashion. Awareness of systems concepts will begin to influence our profession by expanding the therapist-client relationship and increase the practice of more integrated methods.

Table 1-3 Conceptual Model Comparison

Traditional Concepts	Dynamic Systems Concepts
Linear thought process—cause and effect thinking. Basis for our current scientific model.	Circular thought process—ongoing discovery. Questions emerge through process.
Goal and outcome orientation—goals are preset by therapist. Measures of outcomes are predetermined by diagnosis.	Process orientation—goals are dynamic in nature and emerge through treatment process with patient contribution.
Evaluation process separate from treatment.	Constant evaluation—reevaluation dynamic integrated with treatment.
Therapist is the expert and has knowledge to impart to patient.	Innate self-knowledge of patient—therapist becomes facilitator or educator.
Norms establish criteria for comparison to patient.	Individual is unique expression, may or may not fit norms.
Individual is ruled by preset internal determinants or external governing principles.	Individual is dynamically self-organizing in nature.
Patient fits into therapist's worldview. "Tests" accurately reflect reality of situation.	Patient's worldview is primary determinant in expression of dysfunction, may or may not obey our rules.
Hierarchical model—therapist is in superior position relative to patient and therefore in control of situation.	Relational interaction—relationship between therapist and patient is a dynamic interplay.
Therapist treats disease or dysfunction.	Therapist treats patient or host as well as disease.
Reductionism—highly specialized and segmental approach to health care; treat individual body parts.	Holism—relationship between emotion, spirit, mind, and body is interactive and inseparable; treat whole person.
Simplify enormous complexity into manageable units for understanding; sacrifice some possibilities.	Understand complexity of possibilities is infinite and therefore predictable only within certain ranges of probability.

Tenets of Positional Release Technique

The contributions and influence of osteopathy and dynamic systems theory should be clear as we look at the philosophy of Positional Release developed here. The systems perspective may help to integrate these ideas into a cohesive foundation for physical therapy practice in general.

1. *Integrative function of the nervous system.* As organizer and processor of information for an individual's holding and movement patterns, behaviors, responses, history, and cognition, the central and autonomic nervous systems must be considered in all aspects of evaluation and treatment. Positional Release is thought to access the nervous system through manipulation of soft tissues and joints by affecting afferent reduction. Remember the nervous system, sense organs, and skin all arise from the outermost embryonic cells, the ectoderm. Ashley Montagu, in *Touching: The Human Significance of the Skin*, stated, "think and speak of the skin as the external nervous system, an organ system which from its earliest differentiation remains in intimate association with the internal or central nervous system."[16] Therefore, palpation is emphasized with the practice of Positional Release as a tool of evaluation and the primary monitor of patient response during treatment.

2. *Therapist as facilitator or educator.* In one aspect, the therapist using Positional Release serves as an instrument of biofeedback for patients by increasing their awareness of postural and other muscular holding patterns. Once a client becomes aware of the pattern, even on an unconscious level, he or she has a choice to either continue in their old pattern or make a change. The therapist can greatly facilitate this process by taking an "awareness break" or pausing during treatment to ask patients to verbalize the changes they feel. Comparing two legs or two sides of the body is often used. By actively engaging the patient in the process, the feedback loop is completed. With Positional Release, this occurs when getting patient feedback regarding the position of comfort or a change in point tenderness with palpation. Any other methods a therapist can employ to focus the responsibility for change back on the patient also are desirable.

3. *Constant reassessment and reevaluation.* Palpation is a tool by which the therapist can gain a nearly instantaneous and continuous monitor of the patient's response with Positional Release. By developing palpation skills, the tissue changes become more easily perceivable. Other evaluation tools, such as range of motion, postural assessment, or performance of a specific functional task, can be repeated each time the patient is seen. These measures even may need to be reassessed within a given treatment session if a significant change is thought to have occurred.

4. *Honoring the uniqueness of each individual.* It would be more convenient for the therapist if patients would simply obey the rules we learn in school and classes; however, this often is the exception rather than the rule. As each snowflake is unique in nature, so is each person we treat. The complexity of each person's system is vast. There always are unknowns, so expect the unexpected and allow for possibilities that you may not have considered yet.

5. *Innate intelligence of organism.* If we assume innate intelligence governs an organism, it is logical to conclude that the holding and organizational patterns with which they present represent the highest expression of which they are capable at that moment and given certain formative circumstances. When using Positional Release technique, the patient's patterns of presentation are honored, explored, and even exaggerated to ultimately invoke change to a more optimal pattern.

Thomas Hanna, a Feldenkrais® practitioner and author of *Somatics*, distinguished between the "soma," or living body, which is an internal perception of oneself, and the "body," which can be objectively measured by an external perspective.[17] With therapeutic intervention, we can interact with patients only from a "body" or external reference point; however, we must be aware of the "soma" and all that it represents internally to our patients. Their presentation often will give you a clue about their "soma," or internal world. Know that more than a physical or "body" pattern can change with interventions such as Positional Release.

6. *Treating the whole person.* It is important to begin to understand that the physical body is interrelated and connected to other aspects of the self. Factors that influence each person include physical, mental, emotional, spiritual, and social contexts. Practitioners may think they are treating only the physical body, but in fact they are interacting with a system that includes all these complex aspects of the self. Awareness of this fact alone will begin to influence treatment and patient interaction in new ways.

Emotional responses are the most likely to occur and are obvious when they do occur during a treatment session. It is important that we do not negate this or any other expression of inner experience with which the patient may respond. If you do not have training in the psychological field, it is best to simply provide support during the process by being a neutral witness for them. A practitioner who becomes aware of a significant psychological component to the client's somatic dysfunction should consider a referral to a psychotherapist or other professionally trained counselor. However, be aware that this sometimes can be considered, by the patient, a negation of the physical origins of the dysfunction.

7. *Whole body perspective.* It is important to have a treatment perspective that includes the entire body; this is different from treating the entire body in any given session. Avoid tunnel vision and limiting your awareness to only the area(s) of dysfunction. Consider visceral and autonomic responses as well. Begin to think in terms of relationships between various parts of the body. For example, how does the shoulder relate or interact with the pelvis regarding the patient's holding and movement patterns? Positional Release treatment may trigger a response distant to the area of the body currently being treated. Patients often will relate this to you as an unusual sensation or awareness.

8. *Patient-centered therapy.*[18] Remember, from a systems perspective, the patient's presentation and response can take precedence over our scientific knowledge base. While extensive knowledge of anatomy is very useful in learning Positional Release techniques, this is only a starting point in treatment. For example, the individual may have fascial or other components to the dysfunction, usually secondary to trauma, that override the underlying anatomical considerations. Learn to be responsive to individual variations and alter the release or treatment accordingly. To the best of your ability, listen to the patient and keep focused on his or her well being rather than your own agenda.

Summary of Positional Release Treatment Principles

The treatment principles in Positional Release are easy to learn and apply. The following procedural suggestions should provide an introduction to the method or a refresher if you forget a specific release position. More detailed treatment information can be found in Chapters 5, 7, 12, and 17.

- Follow ease of motion.
- Movement is away from pain.
- Approximate origin and insertion of muscle.
- Go away from joint barrier.
- Recreate original position of injury.
- Incorporate the patient's unique structural pattern into release.
- Palpate for softening of tissues.
- Find the balanced point, where all tissues are relaxed.
- Return to a resting position slowly and with support.
- Use isometrics following releases as needed.

References

1. Hoover HV. Fundamentals of technique. In: *Yearbook of the Academy of Applied Osteopathy.* Ann Arbor, MI: Edwards Brothers; 1949:25–41.
2. Greenman PE. *Principles of Manual Medicine.* Baltimore: Williams & Wilkins; 1989.

3. Johnston WL, Friedman HD. *Functional Methods: A Manual for Palpatory Skill Development in Osteopathic Examination and Manipulation of Motor Function.* Indianapolis: American Academy of Osteopathy; 1994.
4. Jones LH, with Kusunose RS, Goering EK. *Jones Strain-CounterStrain.* Boise, ID: Jones Strain-CounterStrain; 1995.
5. Magoun HI. *Osteopathy in the Cranial Field.* 3rd ed. Kirksville, MO: The Journal Printing Co.; 1976.
6. Pfrimmer TC. *Muscles: Your Invisible Bonds.* St. Catharines, ONT: Provoker Press; 1970.
7. Rolf IP. *Rolfing: The Integration of Human Structures.* New York: Harper & Row; 1977.
8. Feldenkrais, M. *Awareness Through Movement: Health Exercises for Personal Growth.* New York: Harper & Row; 1972.
9. Still AT. *Philosophy of Osteopathy.* Newark, OH: American Academy of Osteopathy; 1899.
10. Thelen E. Motor development: A new synthesis. *Am Psychologist.* February 1995;50:79–95.
11. Thelen E, Smith LB. *A Dynamic Systems Approach to the Development of Cognition and Action.* Cambridge, MA: MIT Press/Bradford Books; 1994.
12. Wolf FA. *Taking the Quantum Leap: The New Physics for Non-Scientist.* New York: Perennial Library/Harper & Row; 1989.
13. Capra, F. *The Web of Life.* New York: Anchor Books/Doubleday; 1996.
14. Prigogine I, Stengers I. *Order out of Chaos: Man's New Dialogue with Nature.* Toronto: Bantam Books; 1984.
15. Gleick J. *Chaos: Making a New Science.* New York: Penguin Books; 1987.
16. Montagu A. *Touching: The Human Significance of the Skin.* 3rd ed. New York: Harper & Row; 1986:5.
17. Hanna T. *Somatics: Reawakening the Mind's Control of Movement, Flexibility, and Health.* Reading, MA: Addison-Wesley Publishing Co.; 1988:19–21.
18. Jensen GM, Gwyer J, Hack LM, Shepard KF. *Expertise in Physical Therapy Practice.* Boston: Butterworth–Heinmann; 1999:241–242.

2

Theoretical Foundations

Facilitation

Physical therapists frequently face clinical problems associated with hypertonicity and facilitation of the neuromuscular mechanism. Indirect techniques may offer a solution to a multitude of clinical manifestations of facilitation through afferent reduction. Irvin M. Korr's[1] work often is cited as the theoretical basis for indirect work, which includes Functional technique,[2] Strain-CounterStrain®,[3] and Positional Release technique.[4]

The concepts of the "osteopathic lesion" and the "facilitated segment" first were developed in Korr's "The Neural Basis of the Osteopathic Lesion."[5] In this historical treatise, Korr concluded that,

> *An osteopathic lesion represents a facilitated segment of the spinal cord maintained in that state by impulses of endogenous origin entering the corresponding dorsal root. All structures, receiving efferent nerve fibers from that segment are, therefore, potentially exposed to excessive excitation or inhibition.*[5]

An osteopathic lesion has been defined as a segment of the spinal cord that has a lowered motor reflex threshold. The more severe the dysfunction, the lower is the reflex threshold and the weaker a stimulus required for a response.[6–8] This facilitated or hyperexcitable segment of the cord appears to fire more readily in response to a multitude of stimuli and stresses and therefore can become a "neurological lens which focuses irritation upon that segment."[5] Osteopathic manipulation that promotes relaxation of muscular tension and results in a reduction of afferent impulses bombarding the facilitated segment is thought to break this vicious cycle.[2–5]

This model of facilitation includes higher cortical contributions such as postural, emotional, and environmental stressors, which can add further to a hyperreflexive response.[9] Researchers and clinicians have observed that patients who have underlying facilitation often will be hyperresponsive at the involved spinal levels in situations of even mild stress or trauma, as compared to patients with little to no underlying dysfunction. This early work in osteopathy and physiology established a functional model and a strategy of wholeness that remains pertinent when considering a patient from a systems perspective today.

Somatic Dysfunction

By the 1970s the more comprehensive term *somatic dysfunction* had replaced *osteopathic lesion* in the literature, as it more accurately describes the influence of facilitation on visceral, circulatory, metabolic, and musculoskeletal systems.

> *Somatic dysfunction is defined as an alteration or impairment of function of related components of the somatic system, including skeletal, arthrodial, and myofascial structures; and related vascular, lymphatic, and neural elements.*[10]

Johnson provided further refinement of the research literature on somatic dysfunction by placing a strong emphasis on palpatory diagnosis of segmental spinal dysfunction.[11–13] Four criteria were cited as necessary for making a diagnosis of somatic dysfunction. These include location of tissue texture changes, point tenderness, asymmetry of joint movements, and asymmetry of anatomical landmarks at the site of the dysfunction.[14]

Recent studies involving neuroplasticity and spinal learning supported Korr's concept of the facilitated segment and may help explain the pain, point tenderness, and tissue texture changes seen in somatic dysfunction. For example, in discussing nonspecific low-back pain, Williams suggested that neural pathways can demonstrate increased sensitivity following repetitive postural stress, trauma, and inflammation. He further stated that the spine appears to "learn" or retain a "memory" of previous injuries.[14] This hypothesis, which is supported with scientific research by Woolf[15] and Slosberg,[16] may help explain the continuation of facilitation in segmental somatic dysfunction even after relatively minor tissue or nerve damage. Woolf related that a highly sensitized nervous system can present with spontaneous pain (no stimulus), allodynia (pain with innocuous stimuli), or hyperalgesia.[15] Supporting Woolf's observations, long-term alterations of spinal reflex patterns also have been induced by repetitive noxious peripheral stimulation in animals.[16]

Janda identified muscle imbalance patterns of "postural muscles" that tend to become hypertonic through facilitation and "dynamic muscles" that become hypotonic through inhibition as responses to abnormal afferent input. He further noted that treatment often focuses on regaining range of motion and strength without addressing the underlying cause of these dysfunctions.[17–21] In "Exercise and Somatic Dysfunction," Bookhout[22] also advocated that treatment should address not only the muscle imbalances found but the cause of the abnormal afferent information, be it postural or emotional stressors, faulty movement patterns, excessive physical demands, painful stimuli, or neuromuscular or joint dysfunctions.[17–21,23]

Travell and Simons emphasized the circulatory compromise associated with somatic dysfunction.[24,25] In their research, they determined that local ischemic areas of involved or injured soft tissues are a primary factor in the development and continuation of painful myofascial trigger points. Travell and Simons suggested a direct method of intervention as remedy to vascular insufficiency. However, cadaver studies have shown the importance of positioning in restoring circulatory function. Radiopaque dye almost completely filled the blood vessels when an arm was placed in a Positional Release position for the supraspinatus muscle (flexion, abduction, and external rotation), compared to a neutral position (resting at the side) in which no filling of vessels occured.[26] "Unopposed arterial filling" is suggested also to occur within living tissues during a release hold with Strain-CounterStrain technique.[27]

Current osteopathic literature continues to discuss somatic dysfunction as a possible model for medical conditions of unknown etiology, such as reflex sympathetic dystrophy (RSD). Nelson proposed that RSD may be a manifestation of upper thoracic somatic segmental dysfunction.[28]

More specific aspects of somatic dysfunction now are considered as the theoretical foundations of somatomotor, somatovisceral, and somatoemotional components are explored. Two schools of thought regarding the identification of neurological sensors responsible for continued somatic dysfunction, (proprioceptors or nociceptors) also are discussed.

Proprioceptors or Nociceptors

Several investigators (Korr,[29] Walther,[30] DiGiovanna,[31] and Jones[3]) have hypothesized that the probable source of localized and continued stimulation in somatic dysfunction are the proprioceptors. Jones focused on the role of the proprioceptors, especially the muscle spindles in his work.[3] He hypothesized that the somatic dysfunction occurs not because of the original strain (sudden overloading or overstretching) but because of the body's response to the strain, as in a quick panic-like movement away from the strain. The antagonist, or counterstrained, muscle goes from minimal afferent input at the moment of strain to maximal afferent input as a result of the panic movement out of the strained position. Jones's theory was that this panic movement can override the usual nociceptor response to pain. Therefore, the counterstrained muscle reports that it is strained, even though it actually is shorter than its neutral resting length. This proprioceptive misinformation is thought to continue as a neuromuscular dysfunction until the original position of injury is recreated gently with Strain-CounterStrain. This method requires a slow return to neutral from the release position in a manner that does not surprise the central nervous system (CNS), as did the original panic movement.

Several other authors have suggested nociceptors as a second possible cause of acute local inflammatory responses and restrictions that occur with somatic dysfunction.[4,32,33] These investigators observed that, if the original tissue injury is severe, abrupt, or painful enough, powerful nociceptive (flexor withdrawal) responses may be called into play. It has been suggested that the nociceptive reflexes may be more primary in acute injuries and proprioceptive reflexes may be more primary in chronic conditions.[33] Consider a whiplash injury that typically involves both hyperextension and hyperflexion of the cervical spine, as it demonstrates the layered complexity of possibilities with somatic dysfunction in which all tissues are involved and need to be evaluated. Therefore, treatment should be focused on ease of motion and movement away from pain. This requires treating the most involved and painful layers of tissue first.

In "Nociceptive Considerations in Treating with CounterStrain,"[33] Bailey and Dick commented on the role of both theories and bring back into perspective the patient as a whole system:

> *Probably very few dysfunctional states result from either a purely proprioceptive, or nociceptive response. Both are likely to occur simultaneously. Additional factors such as autonomic responses, other reflexive activities, joint receptor responses, or emotional states must also be accounted for. What predominates is largely a matter of degree, determined by conditions both external and internal to the injured tissues. The symptomatic patient represents the accumulated total of an intricate variety of physiologic responses. Our understanding of such complexity begins at the level of the simplistic neurophysiologic analysis proposed here. It must progress with the incorporation of such concepts into the awareness that our patients are more than a complex collection of reflexes. Human beings represent a gestalt, that is, more than the sum of the parts, and as such cannot be fully comprehended by reductionistic analysis. Realizing this, we are returned to a primary osteopathic tenet that rational therapy is based on an understanding of body unity, self-regulatory mechanisms, and the interrelatedness of structure and function.[33]*

This more inclusive theoretical foundation is consistent with the Positional Release method presented here. By checking both sides of the involved joint, treating what you find, and having a keen awareness of the patient's traumatic and emotional history as well as his or her treatment response, the practitioner can provide more comprehensive intervention.

Somatomotor System

Korr provided a conceptual model for why different manipulative techniques (stretching, shortening, and isometrics) may be effective in the treatment of somatic dysfunction.[29] A high gamma gain or activity can increase afferent input and spindle discharge, as with proprioceptive misinformation that results from traumas such as sudden overloading or overstretching. These events and sequelae can result in greater muscle contraction or resistance to lengthening. The intrafusal-extrafusal fiber disparity increases afferent input, which stimulates the extrafusal fibers to contract the muscle in an effort to quiet the spindle (see Figure 2-1). The gamma system may be giving signals for further muscle contraction, in fact, even when the muscle is shortened beyond its resting length.

Indirect techniques, which favor ease of motion and approximation of involved muscles, can decrease this intrafusal-extrafusal fiber disparity. These techniques are thought to reset and quiet the system by decreasing the afferent input through the gamma loop.

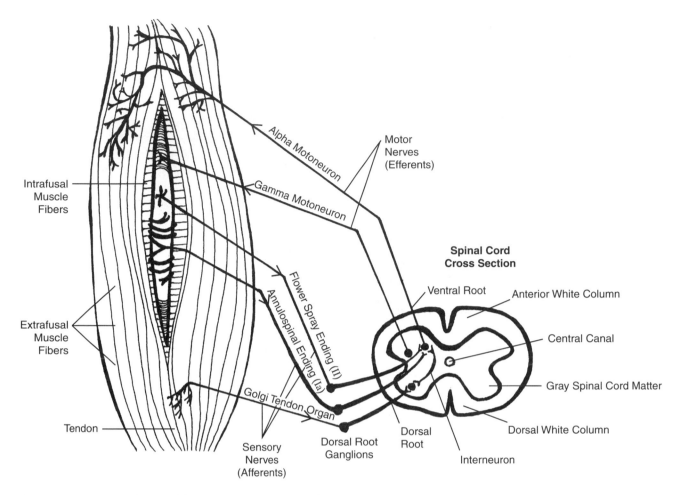

Figure 2-1: Neuromuscular spindle, alpha and gamma motor systems.

The result is a more normal resting length of the muscles and decreased disparity between the intrafusal and extrafusal fibers. This favors lengthening or relaxation of the hypertonic muscle and decreases the facilitation at the target spinal segment. Indirect techniques reduce facilitation by taking the body segment back into or through the original position of trauma slowly with no surprises for the CNS, as the muscle spindle continues to report accurate information throughout the release process.

In techniques that involve stretching, two mechanisms are hypothesized to be responsible for returning the spindles to a more normal gain setting.[29] Stretching a hypertonic muscle bombards the system with afferent input, which somehow may signal the CNS to decrease the gamma discharge. Passive stretching also may cause a strong discharge of the Golgi tendon organ, which may inhibit both the gamma and alpha systems and therefore the intrafusal and extrafusal fibers.

Stretching or movement into a noxious range of motion needs to be avoided, as it elicits an increase in afferent stimulation and sympathetic nerve response.[34] If inflammation is present in a joint, movement within even a normal range of motion stimulates an exaggerated reflex response.[34] It has been discussed that movement, stretching, or strengthening[22] of an effused joint should be avoided. However, if Positional Release technique can be accomplished without triggering a noxious response, it can potentially help reestablish a normal resting length of involved muscles, provide pain relief, and promote tissue healing at an effused joint. Therefore, indirect techniques can be done with more acute injuries in an effort to speed recovery. This also underscores why the patient's pain response should serve as a guideline for all positioning techniques and other therapeutic interventions.

It appears that indirect methods could influence the CNS more directly through afferent reduction than direct methods, which initially increase afferent input into the system. Therefore, being aware of the patient's response to muscle approximation or stretching is very important for the therapist. The goal of resetting the gamma system most likely will not be accomplished if approximation causes further contraction of a hypertonic muscle or if stretching increases tone and tension in the system. Of course, the nature of the somatic dysfunction and the patient response will determine the appropriateness of either treatment technique.

No clinical trials were found in the literature using Strain-CounterStrain, Positional Release, or Functional technique exclusively. Two studies included a combination of manipulative procedures and Strain-CounterStrain.[35,36] Two unpublished studies[37,38] on Positional Release that used outcome measures of range of motion[37] and surface EMG[38] demonstrated no significant differences in these parameters after a single treatment with Positional Release. An unpublished study by Annis found that the addition of Positional Release to a traditional physical therapy protocol increased the range of motion for both straight leg raise and hip abduction in a population of seven preschool-aged children with spastic cerebral palsy.[39] Range of motion increased for all four children in the experimental Positional Release group, after six weeks of 12 or 14 Positional Release treatments on the hamstring and hip adductor muscles. Both straight leg raise and hip abduction range of motion measures increased 17–37%, with the most severely limited children demonstrating the most significant change. No change in range of motion was found in those children in the control group who received traditional physical therapy treatments of stretching. Functional abilities and symmetry between the extremities also improved in the experimental Positional Release group. Given the lack of published studies on this topic, a need for further clinical research on Positional Release is apparent.

Somatovisceral Considerations

The function of visceral organs has been shown to be modulated by either somatosympathetic or somatoparasympathetic reflex activity through stimulation of corresponding somatic afferents in anesthetized lab animals.[40,41] Both supraspinal reflexes involving the medulla oblongata and local spinal reflexes have been established as somatosympathetic reflexes.[42–45] More generalized sympathetic responses to afferent stimulation occur when the CNS is left intact, while spinalized animals have demonstrated a strongly segmental response.[46, 47] Both noxious and innocuous cutaneous stimulation were used most often in these experiments, however, muscular and articular afferent stimulation responses also have been investigated.[48] Sympathetic responses included increased heart rate, cerebral cortical blood flow, adrenal medullary hormonal secretion, and splenic immune function.

It has been documented that part of the facilitation in somatic dysfunction includes overstimulation of sympathetic fibers, which may result in visceral pathology.[49,50] A vicious cycle of irritation may result as the visceral afferents further bombard the anterior horn cells, which in turn increase the somatic dysfunction that causes additional irritation of the viscera. Chronic sympathetic hyperactivity, which may play a role in many varied clinical conditions treated by a multitude of practitioners, often can be overlooked because of the tunnel vision associated with medical specialization.[51] Soft tissue or joint manipulation that reestablishes "coherent proprioceptive patterns" in the facilitated region may break this cyclical pattern of dysfunction.[51]

The regulation of visceral function through physical therapy and acupuncture is the subject of current research, notably in Japan.[52–54] This research substantiated that the sympathetic or parasympathetic efferents that dominate a specific reflex depend on the organ stimulated, the area being stimulated, and the mode of stimulation. Somatically induced reflex responses have been shown to affect not only autonomic visceral function but also hormonal and immune functions in anesthetized and conscious animals. These authors suggest the need for further research before conclusions regarding clinical application can be made.[52–54]

The effects of direct soft tissue manipulation (Rolfing) on increasing parasympathetic function of the pelvis in younger subjects also has been documented.[55,56] These findings are consistent with the common clinical observation of increased bowel sounds during manipulative treatment, representing an increased parasympathetic response of gastric motility.

Researchers also are finding more integration of somatic and visceral function in the higher cortical areas than previously thought.[57–60] The nucleus gracilis appears to be an integration center for visceral and somatic (cutaneous) information that provides input into the ventral posteriolateral nucleus of the thalamus.[57] Visceral information also appears to be processed in the primary somatosensory cortex, with response to visceral stimulation in 13 out of 38 somatosensory neurons.[58] The thalamus also has been shown to play an integrative role in processing visceral pain memories, as stimulation can evoke memories of painful visceral experiences such as angina or labor pain years after the original event occurred.[59,60] These studies reflect a high degree of integration between somatic and visceral input into the CNS, which lends complexity to their previously established autonomic nervous system (ANS) spinal reflex relationship.

Primary visceral or viscerosomatic pain needs to be established as distinct from somatovisceral pain, as important differences between visceral and somatic pain mechanisms are investigated.[61,62] Functional abdominal pain syndromes such as irritable bowel syndrome (IBS) are characterized by the development of an abdominal pain syndrome unrelated to any specific gastrointestinal pathology.[62] Positron emission tomography (PET) studies support a visceral hypersensitivity hypothesis, in which IBS patients have increased awareness of gastrointestinal activity secondary to peripheral or central visceral nociceptive pathways.[63–66] Therefore, IBS is a visceral sensory disorder that involves a facilitated response to stimuli, which may be a visceral manifestation of the facilitated segment. Patients with both IBS and fibromyalgia were found to have somatic hyperalgesia, with lower pain thresholds and higher pain frequency than patients with either IBS only and healthy controls.[67] The effects of stress, anxiety, and other emotional stimuli have been documented to increase IBS symptoms, which points to a central nervous system or brain (mind) dysfunction causal link as well.[68–70]

Somatoemotional Considerations

Research continues to enhance our understanding of the complexities involved in the physiology of emotion. This literature review may underscore the depth of the body-mind and somatoemotional connections, illuminate the necessity for a systems approach to intervention, and highlight the need for practitioners to improve their awareness of these issues with intervention.[71–74]

Emotion no longer is seen as a response to physiological arousal alone; rather it appears that a complex interaction of multiple response systems including the ANS, CNS, endocrine, and somatic motor systems are responsible for emotional experience and expression.[75] Experts describe the "emotional motor system" as a CNS response to a threatening experience that modulates the ANS, decreases sensitivity to pain, and activates the hypothalmic-pituitary-adrenal axis.[70,76] Either an increase or decrease in this emotional motor system can cause symptoms such as altered bowel habits, anxiety, or viscerosomatic hypersensitivity.[70]

Several studies in the literature demonstrate the interconnectedness of somatoemotional-visceral physiology and immune response.[70,77,78] A PET study of normal human subjects whose limbic and paralimbic system structures were probed evoked a wide range of somatic, visceral, and emotional responses, including panic attacks.[77] Common "ill-defined" symptoms observed clinically also were evoked with this limbic-paralimbic stimulation. In another recent study, psychotherapeutic intervention was found to be effective in increasing the natural killer cell activity in patients with malignant melanoma and lymphokine-activated killer cell activity in patients with nonmetastatic breast cancer.[78]

Findings support the prevalence of the comorbidity of somatic dysfunction and psychological disorders, especially with neurological diseases.[79,80] A recent study of 300 consecutive referrals to a neurology outpatient department revealed a significant relationship between emotional disorders and somatic symptoms.[79] Nearly half (47%) of these neurological referrals met the DSM-IV (*Diagnostic and Statistical Manual of Mental Disorders*, fourth edition) criteria for a psychiatric diagnosis (most commonly depressive or anxiety disorders). In contrast to the referrals who did not meet the DSM-IV criteria, these patients had more somatic symptoms and were more disabled in social and physical function. In addition, very few wanted to receive any psychological care. Another study showed that 64% of patients with dissociative disorders met the DSM-III criteria for somatization disorder with an average report of 12.4 somatic symptoms.[80] Nervous system disorders were found in 78.6% of the patients with dissociative disorders, compared to a healthy control group, which had a 21.4% prevalence of nervous system disorders.[80]

The complexity and interrelationship of neuroendocrine interactions in the central and peripheral nervous system continued to be explored and supported by research in the field of psychoneuroimmunology.[81–89] The presence of neurotransmitters and hormones such as serotonin,[81–85] norepinephrine, [86,87] epinephrine,[88] and corticotropin[89] and their receptors sites have been found in skeletal muscle[81,82,85–89] and other soft tissues of the body, including the heart,[87,89] spinal cord,[83,84] and adipose tissues.[87] It is not difficult to see how all body systems, structures, and function could be influenced and modulated by the effects of these neurotransmitters. This and future research may provide some insight into the role of skeletal muscles and other soft tissues during somatoemotional releases that occur during manipulative procedures done in physical therapy practice.

Research in the area of posttraumatic stress disorder (PTSD) is pertinent to physical therapy interventions in general and specifically to the Positional Release technique presented here. Documented symptoms of PTSD include hyperarousal, hypervigilance, exaggerated startle response, sleep disturbances, learning difficulties, avoidance, emotional numbing, alexithymia (the inability of a person to experience, understand, or express their emotions), and the resultant development of somatic disorders, loss of neuromodulation, and affect regulation.[90] Minor stimuli can cause intense emotional reactions or, alternately, cause the individual to emotionally shut down and fail to express emotion externally as he or she develops internal somatic manifestations. The CNS of the individual with PTSD reacts to threatening or nonthreatening stimuli with a conditioned autonomic hyperarousal such that the person no longer can rely on bodily sensations to help discriminate between what actually is or is not threatening.[91] With PTSD there also is a compulsion to repeat, reenact, and reexperience the original traumatic event and an inability to discern the past trauma from present experience.[92]

PTSD commonly is thought to be a response to extreme or severe trauma, such as that sustained in combat,[93–97] natural or other disasters,[98–101] terrorist attacks,[102] and with severe forms of physical, emotional, or sexual abuse.[103,104] However, research has shown that PTSD may follow traumatic events of much lessor proportions such as motor vehicle accidents,[105,106] medical procedures,[107] and myocardial infarcts.[108] It is believed that more than 50% of the U.S. population has been exposed to a potentially life-threatening traumatic event in their lives, and 25% have been exposed to more than one such event.[109] For example, burn and digit amputation patients undergoing rehabilitation were found to have a significantly higher incidence of PTSD and alexithymia than healthy volunteers.[110] These results from the PTSD literature indicate that, in a typical physical therapy practice, the clinician frequently may provide treatment to patients who have some PTSD component to their injury or somatic dysfunction.

Somatization of symptoms is well documented in PTSD, especially in situations when the person is unable to express or process the trauma verbally.[94,97,110–112] Researchers noted that trauma often is stored in somatic memory, expressing itself as an increased physiological stress response that affects ongoing evaluation of sensory stimuli.[111] The trauma usually is organized on a somatosensory level with visual images or physical sensations.

If the individual with PTSD is unable to translate these somatic states into emotional expression following the trauma, physical problems are thought to manifest in a variety of ways; these include depressed immune function and impairment of various organ systems, including the nervous and musculoskeletal systems.[80,112] This emotional trauma or response may be triggered by manipulation of the striated or smooth muscles, which are rich with neurotransmitters and hormones. Emotional expression then may occur when a stimulus such as indirect work actually takes the person back into his or her physical position at the time of the original trauma or otherwise stimulates the client's emotional memory system.

A multitude of factors may contribute to the clinical presentation of individuals with PTSD. The increased state of ANS arousal[113] and somatization that accompanies PTSD can account for the decreased stimuli required to initiate a response in these patients, especially in regards to bodily contact. The physical therapist's touch may become the stimulus for memory processing in patients with any history of trauma.

Awareness of the patient's preexisting psychological traumas could help the practitioner understand a dramatic somatic and emotional response to a relatively minor physical therapy intervention when it occurs. An increased level of responsibility on the part of the physical therapist also should accompany this increased awareness. The clinician needs to provide the patient an environment where he or she feels safe and to lend adequate support during therapy as deemed appropriate.[114] Outside referral to a psychological support person also should be considered. According to Van der Kolk, a PTSD expert,

> Exploring the trauma for its own sake has no therapeutic benefits unless it becomes attached to other experiences, such as feeling understood, being safe, feeling physically strong and capable, or being able to empathize with and help fellow sufferers.[112]

Systems Theory

The word *system* is derived from the Greek word *synhistanai*, which means "to place together."[115] A system denotes the integrated whole of both living organisms and social or ecological systems. *Systems thinking* emphasizes relationship among the parts of a system as the primary organizing force. The individual parts of a system are understood within the context of the larger whole, so that the whole becomes greater than just the sum of its parts.

Physicist Fritjof Capra provides an extensive historical perspective of the evolution of systems theory and the "paradigm shift" that it implies, in several of his writings, including *The Turning Point*, "The Concept of Paradigm and Paradigm Shift," and *The Web of Life*.[116–118] According to Capra, in the early 1900s, Alexander Bogdanov, a little known Russian medical researcher, developed a theory of the organizing principles operating in living and nonliving systems, called *tektology*, or "the science of structures."[119]

The field of organismic biology developed during the early 20th century as the study of cell structure turned toward the organizing, coordinating, and integrative functions of cell life. Ludwig von Bertalanffy, an Australian organismic biologist, developed his "general systems theory" in the 1930s, which often is thought to be the first comprehensive theoretical framework for living systems.[120] By the 1930s, physiologist Walter Cannon also had refined the concepts of homeostasis or dynamic self-regulation of organisms.[121]

Systems theory may have its origins in the fields of biology and physiology,[120,121] but system thinking has spread to many fields of study, including sociology, psychology, ecology, mathematics, organizational planning, and management. By the 1940s, the field of cybernetics evolved, as mathematicians, social scientists, engineers, and neuroscientists developed the system ideas of dynamic patterns, feedback loops, self-regulation, and self-organization.[122]

Discovery of these communication and feedback patterns originating in cybernetics led social scientists, such as Margaret Mead and Gregory Bateson, to lend their vast contributions to systems thinking. As a trained anthropologist, Bateson wrote the pioneering book, *Mind and Nature: A Necessary Unity*, which develops a model of the underlying unity of humankind and the universe.[123] He developed ideas of binocular rather than monocular vision and suggested that multiple levels of understanding are accessible within any given system. He also explored the commonality between the natural world and our mental processes and redefined the *mind* from this perspective. Bateson headed a research project that attempted to classify different levels of communication including levels of meaning, levels of logical type, and levels of learning. This extremely innovative research included such diversity as study of animal behavior, play, hypnosis, paradoxes, and the communication of schizophrenics in family systems.[124]

The field of psychology has been deeply affected by systems thinking, as represented by family systems therapy and Gestalt psychology. Bateson's earlier research on families with a schizophrenic member were later expanded on by a number of psychiatrists and psychologists, including the originator of family systems theory, Murry Bowen, M.D.[125] Bowen theory is based on the assumptions that an individual's emotional function must be studied in context with their relational systems, which are rooted in nature and therefore involve relationship to all life.[125,126] Gestalt psychology originated in Germany during the 1920s, concurrent with, yet independent of, the rise of organismic biology.[127] This therapeutic approach explores the experiential process of the individual from multiple perspectives and emphasizes the integrated whole, including body work and body awareness.[128]

The field of ecology, which also emerged from the influence of organismic biology, includes the study of all natural ecosystems such as plant and animal communities, as well as issues of concern to human communities.[129] Arne Naess a Norwegian philosopher, founded the school of "deep ecology," which values all living things and focuses on the network of interconnections and the interdependence between its interrelated parts.[130] This is compared to "shallow ecology," which is human centered and views the world as a collection of separate and isolated objects. The evolution of ecocentric, or earth-centered, values and ethics is at the core of deep ecology and the paradigm shift.

Systems influence in the field of mathematics, commonly referred to as *mathematics of complexity*, is an extremely important development of 20th century science.[118] Dynamical systems theory or nonlinear dynamics has emerged as a result of the availability of new mathematical and computerized tools.[131] These mathematical advances allow for patterns of highly complex systems, from a broad range of fields, to be mapped and understood in new ways. New insights, observations, and discoveries such as chaos theory, have resulted from the availability of mathematics of complexity or dynamical systems theory.[132]

The widespread influence of systems thinking in the 20th century is evident by this review from many fields of endeavor. Until recently, the fields of medicine and physical therapy have been somewhat slower to embrace a systems perspective in patient care. However, medical journal articles from a broad spectrum of practitioners call for a paradigm shift, especially regarding the mind-body duality issue.[14,133–139] This may be indicative of a changing attitude in mainstream medicine and a growing movement toward a more integrative systems perspective of health care. It appears evident that our profession and our patients could benefit greatly from a systems perspective in the treatment of patients with orthopedic, neurological, and cardiopulmonary disorders.

Physics and a Systems Perspective

Classic Newtonian physics, which views the universe from the perspective of a solid, mechanical, and deterministic model, has dominated science and philosophy since the 1600s. Newton's theories are based on a foundation of absolute space and time, where time is linear, from past to present to future, and matter always is conserved and essentially passive.[140] In classic physics, the world is described objectively according to formulas of speed, position, and motion. Everything material and nonmaterial is predictable and predetermined, the future is a consequence of the past, in Newton's clock-like machine.[141]

Classic mechanical thinking is useful when describing the motion of everyday objects. According to Newtonian physics, the material world is a collection of solid objects, which move along straight lines propelled by fixed laws of motion. To the extent that our universe and our bodies conform to this fixed, geometric, and mechanical model, it may be useful to consider Newton's third law of motion, when thinking about trauma and Positional Release technique. The law reads, "if a body A exerts a force F on a second body B, then that body B will exert on body A an oppositely directed force of magnitude equal to F."[142] This more commonly is referred to as "for every action there is an equal and opposite reaction."[142] (See the Chapter 5 section on fascial strain patterns and force vectors for treatment application of Newton's law.)

In the early 1900s, the foundation of the scientific world began to shift, when new experiments began to question and challenge the Newtonian worldview. New theories emerged, which explored the macrocosmic and microcosmic universe. These included Einstein's theory of relativity, which explored time and space relationships, as well as quantum mechanics theory, developed by Heisenberg, Planck, Bohr, and others, which began to probe the subatomic world.[141]

Max Planck solved the "black body radiation" problem by explaining why steel and lava become red hot and then white when heated to high temperatures. His discovery was that light, which was thought to be a wave, actually could be divided into "quanta" and act like a particle. Planck developed a formula—energy (E) equals the frequency of the light emitted (f) times a constant (h)[140]—that described the relationship between the frequency of light and the energy needed to produce the light. Planck's constant turned out to be a very tiny number ($h = 6.5 \times 10^{-27}$), which accounts for why we never observe these quantum effects in everyday life.[143] The development of quantum theory left researchers attempting to reconcile why our world, which appears solid and continuous, actually is made of building blocks that are fundamentally discontinuous and behave by jumping or leaping from one quantum level to another.

Neils Bohr developed the Bohr principle of complementarity, which implies that there is no reality until that reality is perceived.[141] The complementary principle appears to challenge the assumption that observations verify an existing reality. The mere act of observation has been shown to disturb electron activity, as the subatomic particles often behave according to the outcome expected by the observer. The premise here is that nature is dualistic, and the more we determine one complement (or side of reality), the less is known about the other complement or reality base. According to Wolf, "There is, instead, one unbroken wholeness that appears paradoxical as soon as we observers attempt to analyze it. We can't help but disrupt the universe in our efforts to take things apart."[141] These findings in quantum physics appear to verify a systems approach to health care and call into question the premise of truly being able to objectify outcome data.

David Bohm, in *Wholeness and the Implicate Order*, developed the idea of wholeness from a quantum physics perspective.[144] He described the totality of existence, including matter and consciousness, as an interconnected and interrelated unbroken whole. Bohm discussed the widespread fragmentation that currently rules every aspect of our lives, including external social, political, economic, racial, and religious separations and internal psychological and physical separations, supported and reinforced by medical specialties.

So, what is the relevance of all this new physics to the content of this book, apart from the obvious implications these revelations have on science and medicine as a whole? The concepts of quantum physics support the dynamic systems perspective that subscribes to wholeness and includes all influences significant to the system in question. This science also is entirely consistent with the osteopathic worldview that is the basis for Positional Release and most manual therapy techniques. Thus, relationships within the individual's system (i.e., visceral, sympathetic, and emotional components) as well as relationships external to that system (the therapist, the environment, and social contexts) appear extremely relevant to treatment selection, progression, and outcomes. The nature of patient handling with Positional Release implies respect for these internal and external factors.

Admittedly, it may be difficult to consider both Newtonian and quantum physics simultaneously during physical therapy evaluation and intervention. Newton's contribution to science is immense; however, his "playing field" was limited. It now is recognized that humans are part of a universe that is much more expansive, interesting, and dynamically alive. This probing has lead to bigger questions for physicists; the universe remains as intriguing, yet unfathomable, and cloaked in paradox, as are we.[118,145–147] Science took a strange turn in the early 1900s that has led us back to the mysteries of life.

Nonlinear Dynamics

Dynamical systems theory, or nonlinear dynamics, provides a mathematical means to study a wide array of complex systems, such as those found in nature or in the human body. Computer advancements in the 1970s increased the scientist's capacity to study large amounts of data over time and simulate conditions using Newtonian physics. Scientists discovered that extremely small changes in initial conditions resulted in significant changes in outcome patterns. This came to be known as *sensitivity to original conditions* or the *butterfly effect,* such that, with all other conditions being equal, the flapping of a butterfly's wing will result in a different outcome of data.[148]

The first chaotic system described was Edward Lorenz's waterwheel, which demonstrates infinite complexity within certain bounds. "Nature forms patterns. Some are orderly in space but disorderly in time, others orderly in time but disorderly in space. Some patterns are fractal, exhibiting structures self-similar in scale. Others give rise to steady states or oscillating ones."[148] J. Gleick saw the essence of chaos as, "a delicate balance between forces of stability and instability."[148] The dynamic model that emerges is one of data collection that yields shapes, which change in space and time.

Although chaos theory still is in its infancy, it has developed widespread appeal as a means of predicting patterns of complex systems in nature that have the commonality of seemingly erratic, irregular, and discontinuous behavior. Due to the global nature of systems being explored, chaos theory has attracted a cross-disciplinary collection of scientists, such as mathematicians, physicists, chemists, biologists, ecologists, meteorologists, and physiologists all seeking to explore the "universal behavior of complexity."[148] Research into chaos theory appears to be a natural fit for the complex and dynamic systems of the human body.

Chaos theory explores the complex world of nonlinear equations, which best describe most occurrences in our natural world. Few events follow the cause-effect linear equation model, where increasing the force results in an ever-rising increase in outcome or response. There are limits to the increasing effects. Nonlinear relationships are the result of feedback loops, both positive and negative, within the system. For example, consider these equations as representing the ideal amount of weight used in a strengthening program. Increasing the resistance or poundage will result in increased strength up to a certain point (a linear relationship), but the resistance cannot continue to be increased indefinitely without detrimental effects. At a certain point, further increase in poundage will have an inverse effect on strength (a nonlinear relationship). See Figure 2-2 for a comparison of a familiar linear equation and a simple nonlinear equation.

By the 1980s, scientists began to investigate the complex and dynamic systems of the human body from a chaos perspective. Study of heart rhythms has dominated the chaos theory research done on the human body. Normal healthy cardiac rhythm is periodic or predictably repeatable. Unstable rhythmical states of the heart, such as tachycardia and fibrillation, are chaotic patterns that represent a diseased state with potentially

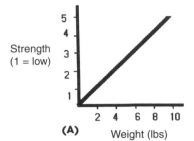

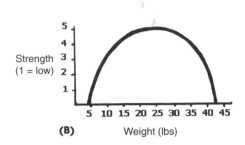

Figure 2-2: Comparison of linear (A) and nonlinear equations (B).

fatal consequences.[149,150] In fibrillation, the normal periodic wave forms break up so the heart never fully relaxes or fully contracts and, therefore, cannot pump blood.

Research on brain waves has demonstrated an opposite finding. A chaotic pattern actually represents health in brain function. Normal brain function is more random and chaotic in nature. During an epileptic seizure, brain waves become too repetitive or patterned in a periodic phase.[151,152]

If health in cardiac function is a periodic pattern and health in brain function is a chaotic pattern, what represents a healthy pattern in the neuromuscular system? A person who has highly patterned movement behavior (periodic pattern) presents a great deal of stability and predictability of motion. A person who has more random or chaotic movement behavior presents a more variable and flexible pattern of motion with less predictability. In the extreme, either of these patterns may represent a pathological or dysfunctional neuromuscular state. As physical therapists, we need to move the highly patterned person into more freedom and choice of movement and the highly flexible person into a more stable pattern of function.

Kauffman described a healthy adaptive system as one that resides at the edge of chaos.[153] From this perspective the system is able to adapt or move into either pattern (periodic-stability or chaotic-flexibility) based on demand for function and environmental circumstances. This ability to function in a relatively high degree of chaos with a multiplicity of movement choices and yet have the potentiality to isolate specific patterns of movement to perform a given function appears ideal when considering neuromuscular patterns.

In dynamic, complex systems, attractors represent a stable state to which motions tend to return. A pendulum is used to demonstrate this concept of attractors. A pendulum will swing when set in motion but gradually will lose energy to friction until it reaches its attractor, a steady state in this case of no motion at the center of its trajectory. If the pendulum is swinging in a frictionless system, a periodic pattern or perfectly predictable back and forth oscillation will occur. In this case, the attractor is a circle and the stable state is a time-dependent motion. This periodic pattern is highly stable and predictable, as illustrated in Figure 2-3.

If this predictable one pendulum system is expanded to include two attached pendulums, an increasingly complex pattern evolves. Movement of the coupled pendulums can result in a more complex periodic pattern or a chaotic pattern, depending on several factors including the strength of the attraction between the two pendulums. If the pendulums become somewhat synchronized the result will be more a complex periodic pattern, as illustrated in Figure 2-4. Here, the attractor still causes a circular pattern, but with more variation of possibility due to the interaction of two pendulums. A chaotic pattern may develop if the coupling strength is weaker and the interactive pattern becomes less organized and predictable. This dynamic pattern of chaos is illustrated in Figure 2-5 with its "strange attractor." In this case, the movement has increased variability, has less stability, and is less predictable than previously. The chaotic pattern that develops (in the pendulums' motion) results from the interrelationship of the pendulums and can be predicted only within a range of possibilities.

The pendulum example may have application to the physical structure and function of the human body, especially when considering the neuromuscular and skeletal com-

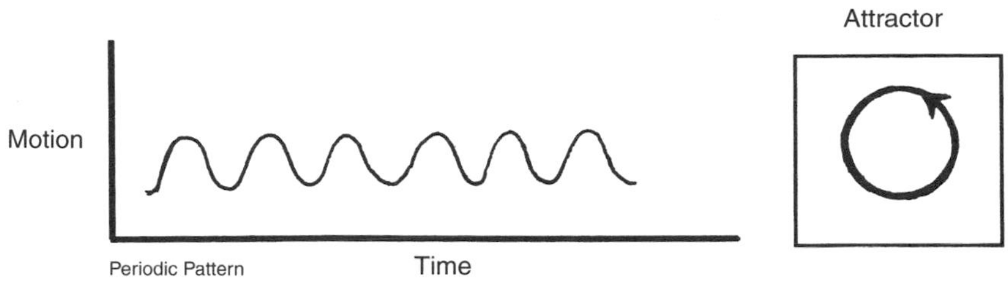

Figure 2-3: Periodic pattern with stable attractor.

Figure 2-4: Intermediate pattern with attractor.

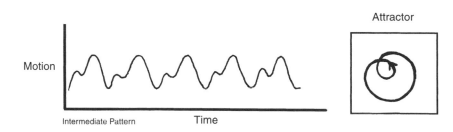

Figure 2-5: Dynamic chaotic pattern with strange attractor.

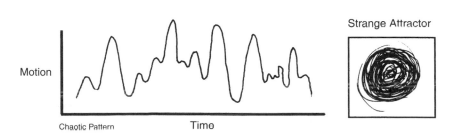

ponents commonly treated by physical therapists. Healthy functioning results when soft tissues and bony relationships function primarily in homeostasis with one another and other body systems, with optimal conditions of friction, gravity, posture, muscle balance, and emotional well-being. With disease states involving systemic, metabolic, hormonal, or emotional disturbances or with injury, inflammation, disuse, or other insults, the soft and bony tissues of the body may respond by expressing of chaotic or disturbed patterns of dysfunction and pathology. When all systems of the body function in a harmonious fashion, health and wellness result.

Patient outcomes may be improved significantly by using Positional Release technique in a timely and appropriate intervention after injury, trauma, or surgery. The "butterfly effect" must be kept in mind when considering the advantages of an indirect manual intervention, as minor changes in initial conditions can result in significant differences in the pattern that develops in a system, be it functional or dysfunctional. Optimal conditions for healing can be established early in treatment by releasing the neuromuscular dysfunction, restoring normal muscle length, and improving circulatory function. Therefore, the secondary effects of neural and circulatory imbalance such as inflammation, edema, ischemia, visceral involvement, and chronic pain syndromes will not be as likely to develop.

References

1. Peterson B., ed. *The Collected Papers of Irvin M. Korr.* Indianapolis: American Academy of Osteopathy; 1979.
2. Johnston WL, Friedman HD. *Functional Methods: A Manual for Palpatory Skill Development in Osteopathic Examination and Manipulation of Motor Function.* Indianapolis: American Academy of Osteopathy; 1994.

3. Jones LH with Kusunose RS, Goering EK. *Jones Strain-CounterStrain.* Boise, ID: Jones Strain-CounterStrain; 1995.

4. Chaitow L. *Positional Release Techniques: Advanced Soft Tissue Techniques.* New York: Churchill Livingstone; 1996:12–13.

5. Korr IM. The neural basis of the osteopathic lesion. *JAOA.* 1947;47:191–198.

6. Denslow JS, Clough GH. Reflex activity in spinal extensors. *J Neurophysiology.* 1941;4:430–437.

7. Denslow JS, Hassett CC. Central excitatory state associated with postural abnormalities. *J Neurophysiology.* 1942;5:393–402.

8. Denslow JS. Analysis of variability of spinal reflex thresholds. *J Neurophysiology.* 1944;7:207-215.

9. Denslow JS, Korr IM, Krems AD. Quantitative studies of chronic facilitation in human motoneuron pools. *Am J. Physiology.* 1947;105:229–238.

10. Bourdillon JF, Day EA, Bookhout MR. *Spinal Manipulation.* 5th ed. Oxford, England: Butterworth–Heinemann; 1992.

11. Johnston WL, Allan BR, Hendra JL, Neff DR, et al. Interexaminer study of palpation in detecting location of spinal segmental dysfunction. *JAOA.* 1983;82:839–845.

12. Johnston WL. Segmental definition: Part I. A focal point for diagnosis of somatic dysfunction. *JAOA.* 1988;88:99–105.

13. Johnston WL. Segmental definition: Part II. Application of an indirect method in osteopathic manipulative treatment. *JAOA.* 1988;88:211–217.

14. Williams N. Managing back pain in general practice—Is osteopathy the new paradigm? *Br J of Gen Practice.* 1997;47:653–655.

15. Woolf CJ. Recent advances in the pathophysiology of acute pain. *Br J Anaesth.* 1989;63:139–146.

16. Slosberg M. Spinal learning: Central modulation of pain processing and long-term alteration of interneuronal excitability as a result of nociceptive peripheral input. *J of Manipulation & Physiological Ther.* 1990;13:326–336.

17. Janda V. Muscles, central nervous motor regulation and back problems. In: Korr IM, ed. *The Neurological Mechanisms in Manipulative Therapy.* New York: Plenum Press; 1977:27.

18. Janda V. Muscles as a pathogenic factor in back pain. In: *The Treatment of Patients.* Proceedings International Federation of Orthopaedic Manipulative Therapists, fourth conference, Christchurch, New Zealand; 1980:1.

19. Janda V. Muscle weakness and inhibition (pseudoparesis) in back pain syndrome. In: Grieve G, ed. *Modern Manual Therapy of the Vertebral Column.* New York: Churchill-Livingstone; 1986:197.

20. Jull GA, Janda V. Muscles and motor control in low back pain: Assessment and management. In: Twomey LT, Taylor JR, eds. *Physical Therapy of the Low Back.* New York: Churchill-Livingstone; 1987:253.

21. Janda V. Muscles and motor control in cervicogenic disorders: Assessment and management. In: Grant R, ed. *Modern Manual Therapy of the Vertebral Column.* New York: Churchill-Livingstone; 1986:197.

22. Bookhout MR. Exercise and somatic dysfunction. *Physical Medicine and Rehabilitation Clinics of North America.* 1996;7:845–862.

23. Janda V. Treatment of chronic back pain. *J of Manual Medicine.* 1992;6:166.

24. Travell J, Simons D. *Myofascial pain and dysfunction,* Vol 1. Baltimore: Williams & Wilkins; 1983.

25. Travell J, Simons D. *Myofascial Pain and Dysfunction,* Vol 2. Baltimore: Williams & Wilkins; 1992.

26. Rathburn J, Macnab I. Microvascular pattern at the rotator cuff. *Bone and Joint Surgery.* 1970;52:540–553.

27. Jacobson E, et al. Shoulder pain and repetition strain injury. *JAOA.* 1989;89:1037–1045.

28. Nelson KE. Osteopathic medical considerations of reflex sympathetic dystrophy. *JAOA.* 1997;97:286–289.

29. Korr IM. Proprioceptors and somatic dysfunction. *JAOA.* 1975;74:638–650.

30. Walther D. *Applied Kinesiology.* Pueblo, CO: SDC Systems; 1988.

31. DiGiovanna E. *An Osteopathic Approach to Diagnosis and Treatment.* Philadelphia: Lippincott; 1991.

32. Van Buskirk RL. Nociceptive reflexes and the somatic dysfunction: A model. *JAOA.* 1990;90:792–809.

33. Bailey M, Dick L. Nociceptive considerations in treating with CounterStrain. *JAOA.* 1992;92:334–341.

34. Sato A, Sato Y, Schmidt RF. Catecholamine secretion and adrenal nerve activity in response to movements of normal and inflamed knee joints in cats. *J Physiolo (Lond)*. 1986;375:611–624.

35. Walko EJ, Janouschek C. Effects of osteopathic manipulative treatment in patients with cervicothoracic pain: Pilot study using thermography. *JAOA*. 1994;94:135–141.

36. Radjieski JM, Lumley MA, Cantieri MS. Effect of osteopathic manipulative treatment on length of stay for pancreatitis: A randomized pilot study. *JAOA*. 1998;98:264–272.

37. Stikeleather JS. *Effects of Positional Release on Cervical Range of Motion* [masters thesis]. Indianapolis: University of Indianapolis, 1989.

38. Deig DK. *The Effects of Positional Release and Stretching on Surface EMG Activity of Upper Trapezius Muscles* [masters thesis]. Indianapolis: University of Indianapolis, 1994.

39. Annis GR. *The Effects of Positional Release on Lower Extremity Range of Motion of Children with Spastic Cerebral Palsy* [masters thesis]. Indianapolis: University of Indianapolis, 1988.

40. Koizumi K, Brooks C McC. The integration of autonomic system reactions: A discussion of autonomic reflexes, their control and their association with somatic reactions. *Rev Physiol. Biochem. Pharmacol.* 1972;67:1–68.

41. Sato A, Schmidt RF. Somatosympathetic reflexes: Afferent fibers, central pathways, discharge characteristics. *Physiol. Rev.* 1973;53:916–947.

42. Alexander RS. Tonic and reflex functions of medullary sympathetic cardiovascular centers. *J. Neurophysiol.*1946;9:205–217.

43. Coote JH, Downman CBB. Central pathways of some autonomic reflex discharges. *J Physiol (Lond.).* 1966;183:714–729.

44. Franz DN, Evans MH, Perl ER. Characteristics of viscerosympathetic reflexes in the spinal cat. *Am. J. Physiol.* 1966;211:1292–1298.

45. Sato A, Tsushima N, Fujimori B. Reflex potentials of lumbar sympathetic trunk with sciatic nerve stimulation in cats. *Jpn. J. Physiol.* 1965;15:532–539.

46. Sato A, Schmidt RF. Muscle and cutaneous afferents evoking sympathetic reflexes. *Brain Res.* 1966;2:399–401.

47. Sato A, Schmidt RF. Spinal and supraspinal components of the reflex discharges into lumbar and thoracic white rami. *J Physiol (Lond.).* 1971;212;839–850.

48. Sato A, Schmidt RF. The modulation of visceral functions by somatic afferent activity. *Jpn. J. Physiol.* 1987;37(1):1–17.

49. Korr IM, Wright HM, Thomas PE. Effects of experimental myofascial insults on cutaneous patterns of sympathetic activity in man. *J. Neural Transmission.* 1962;23:330–355.

50. Korr IM, Wright IIM, Chace JA. Cutaneous patterns of sympathetic activity in clinical abnormalities of the musculoskeletal system. *J. Neural Transmission.* 1964;25:589–606.

51. Korr IM, ed. *The Neurobiologic Mechanisms in Manipulative Therapy; Sustained Sympathicotonia as a Factor in Disease.* New York: Plenum Publishing; 1978:229–268.

52. Sato A. Somatovisceral reflexes. *J. Manipulative Physiol Ther.* 1995;18:597–602.

53. Sato A. Neural mechanisms of autonomic responses elicited by somatic sensory stimulation. *Neurosci Behav Physiol.* 1997;27:610–621.

54. Kimura A, Sato A. Somatic regulation of autonomic functions in anesthetized animals—Neural mechanisms of physical therapy including acupuncture. *Jpn J Vet Res.* 1997; 45:137–145.

55. Cottingham JT, Porges SW, Lyon T. Effects of soft tissue mobilization (Rolfing pelvic lift) on parasympathetic tone in two age groups. *Phys Ther.* 1988;68:352–356.

56. Cottingham JT, Porges SW, Richmond K. Shifts in pelvic inclination angle and parasympathetic tone produced by Rolfing soft tissue manipulation. *Phys Ther.* 1988;68:1364–1370.

57. Al-Chaer ED, Westlund KN, Willis WD. Nucleus gracilis: an integrator for visceral and somatic information. *J Neurophysiol.* 1997;78:521–527.

58. Bruggermann J, Shi T, Apkarian AV. Viscero-somatic neurons in the primary somatosensory cortex (SI) of the squirrel monkey. *Brain Res.* 1997;756:297–300.

59. Lenz FA, Gracely RH, Hope EJ, et al. The sensation of angina can be evoked by stimulation of the human thalamus. *Pain.* 1994;59:119–125.

60. Davis KD, Tasker RR, Kiss ZHT, Hutchison WD, Dostrovsky JO. Visceral pain evoked by thalmic microstimulation in humans. *Neuro Report.* 1995;6:369–374.

61. McMahon SB. Are there fundamental differences in the peripheral mechanisms of visceral and somatic pain? *Behav Brain Sci.* 1997;20:381–391;discussion 435–513.

62. Cervero F, Laird JM. Visceral Pain. *Lancet.* 1999;353:2145–2148.

63. Mayer EA, Raybould HE. Role of visceral afferent mechanism in functional bowel disorders. *Gastroenterology.* 1990;99:1688–1704.

64. Lembo T, Munakata J, Mertz H, et al. Evidence for the hypersensitivity of lumbar splanchnic afferents in irritable bowel syndrome. *Gastroenterology.* 1994;107:1686–1696.

65. Accarino AM, Azpiroz F, Malagelada J-R. Selective dysfunction of mechanosensitive intestinal afferents in irritable bowel syndrome. *Gastroenterology.* 1995;108:636–643.

66. Naliboff BD, Muranaka M, Fullerton S, et al. Evidence for two distinct perceptual alterations in irritable bowel syndrome. *Gut.* 1997;41:505–512.

67. Chang L. Differences in somatic perception in female patients with irritable bowel syndrome with and without fibromyalgia. *Pain.* 1999;84:297–307.

68. Fukudo S, Muranaka M, Nomura T, Satake M. Brain-gut interactions in irritable bowel syndrome: physiological and psychological aspect. *Nippon Rinsho.* 1992;50:2703–2711.

69. Anton PA. Stress and mind-body impact on the course of inflammatory bowel diseases. *Semin Gastrointest Dis.* 1999;10:14–19.

70. Mayer EA. Emerging disease model for functional gastrointestinal disorders. *Am J Med.* 1999;107:12S–19S.

71. Wallace ER. Mind-body and the future of psychiatry. *J Med Philos.* 1990;15:41–73.

72. Rossi EL. The psychobiology of mind-body communication: The complex, self-organizing field of information transduction. *Biosystems.* 1996;38:199–206.

73. Goodman A. Organic unity theory: an integrative mind-body theory for psychiatry. *Theor Med.* 1997;18:357–378.

74. Astin JA, Shapiro SL, Lee RA, Shapiro DH Jr. The construct of control in mind-body medicine: Implications for health care. *Altern Ther Health Med.* 1999;5:42–47.

75. Bauer RM. Physiologic measures of emotion. *J Clin Neurophysiol.* 1998;15:388–396.

76. Saper CB. Role of the cerebral cortex and striatum in emotional motor response. *Prog Brain Res.* 1996;107:537–550.

77. Servan-Schreiber D, Perlstein WM, Cohen JD, Mintun M. Selective pharmacological activation of limbic structures in human volunteers: A positron emission tomography study. *J Neuropsychiatry Clin Neurosci.* 1998;10:148–159.

78. Greer S. Mind-body research in psychooncology. *Adv Mind Body Med.* 1999;15:236–244.

79. Carson AJ. Neurological disease, emotional disorder, and disability: They are related: A study of 300 consecutive new referrals to a neurology outpatient department. *J Neurol Neurosurg Psychiatry.* 2000;68:202–206.

80. Saxe GN, Chinman G, Berkowitz R, Hall K, et al. Somatization in patients with dissociative disorders. *Am J Psychiatry.* 1994;151:1329–1334.

81. Guillet-Deniau I, Burnol AF, Girard J. Identification and localization of a skeletal muscle serotonic 5-HT2A receptor coupled to the Jak/STAT pathway. *J Biol Chem.* 1997;272:14825–14829.

82. Wappler F, Scholz J, Von Richthofen V, Fiege M, et al. Attenuation of serotonin-induced contractures in skeletal muscle from malignant hyperthermia-susceptible patients with dantrolene. *Acta Anaesthesiol Scand.* 1997;41:1312–1318.

83. Jankowska E, Lackberg ZS, Dyrehag LE. Effects of monoamines on transmission from group II muscle afferents in sacral segments in the cat. *Eur J Neurosci.* 1994;6:1058–1061.

84. Bervoets K, Rivet JM, Millan MJ. 5-HT sub (1A) receptors and the tail-flick response: IV. Spinally localized 5-HT sub (1A) receptors postsynaptic to serotoninergic neurones mediate spontaneous tail-flicks in the rat. *J Pharmacology & Exp Therap.* 1993;264:95–104.

85. Hindle AT, Hopkins PM. 5-Hydroxytryptamine potentiates post-tetanic twitch responses in the rat phrenic nerve diaphragm preparation. *Eur J Anaesthesiol.* 1998;15:216–223.

86. Powers SK, Wade M, Criswell D, Herb RA, et al. Role of beta-adrenergic mechanisms in exercise training-induced metabolic changes in respiratory and locomotor muscle. *Int J Sports Med.* 1995;16:13–18.

87. Chamberlain PD, Jennings KH, Paul F, Cordell J, et al. The tissue distribution of the human beta3-adrenoceptor studied using a momoclonal antibody: Direct evidence of the beta3-adrenoceptor in human adipose tissue, atrium and skeletal muscle. *Int J Obes Relat Metab Disord.* 1999;23:1057–1065.

88. Niklasson M, Holmang A, Lonnroth P. Induction of rat muscle insulin resistance by epinephrine is accompanied by increased interstitial glucose and lactate concentrations. *Diabetologia.* 1998;41:1467–1473.

89. Heldwein KA, Duncan JE, Stenzel P, Rittenberg MB, et al. Endotoxin regulates corticotropin-releasing hormone receptor 2 in heart and skeletal muscle. *Mol Cell Endocrinol.* 1997;131:167–172.

90. Van der Kolk BA, Fisler RE. The biologic basis of posttraumatic stress. *Prim Care.* 1993;20:417–432.

91. Krystal H. Trauma and affects. *Psychoanalytic Study of the Child.* 1978;33:81–116.

92. Van der Kolk BA. The compulsion to repeat the trauma. Re-enactment, revictimization, and masochism. *Psychiatr Clin North Am.* 1989;12:389–411.

93. Figley CR. *Stress Disorders among Vietnam Veterans.* New York: Brunner/Mazel, 1978.

94. Solomon Z. Somatic complaints, stress reaction and PTSD: A three year follow-up. *Behavioral Med.* 1988;14:179–186.
95. Solomon Z. Characteristic psychiatric symptomatology in PTSD: A three year follow-up. *Psychological Medicine.* 1989;19:927–936.
96. Buydens-Branchey L, Noumair D, Branchey M. Duration and intensity of combat exposure and posttraumatic stress disorders among Vietnam veterans. *J Nerv Ment Dis.* 1990;178:582–587.
97. Pavlovic S, Sinanovic O. Somatization in posttraumatic stress disorders in soldiers during the war in Bosnia-Herzegovina. *Med Arch.* 1999;53:145–149.
98. Koopman C, Classen C, Cardena E, Spiegel D. When disaster strikes, acute stress disorder may follow. *J of Traumatic Stress.* 1995;8:29–46.
99. Koopman C, Classen C, Spiegel D. Predictors of posttraumatic stress symptoms among survivors of the Oakland/Berkeley, California, firestorm *Am J Psychiatry.* 1994;151:888–894.
100. McFarlane AC. Stress and disaster. In: Hobfa SE, deVries MW, eds. *Extreme Stress and Communities.* Dordrecht, the Netherlands: Kluwer: 1995.
101. Weisaeth L. The stressor and the posttraumatic stress syndrome after an industrial disaster. *Acta Psychiatrica Scandinavica.* 1989;80:25–37.
102. Shalev AY. Posttraumatic stress disorder among injured survivors of a terrorist attack: Predictive value of early intrusion and avoidance symptoms. *J Nervous and Mental Disease.* 1992;180:505–509.
103. Ackerman PT, Newton JE, McPherson WB, Jones JG, et al. Prevalence of posttraumatic stress disorder and other psychiatric diagnoses in three groups of abused children (sexual, physical and both). *Child Abuse & Neglect.* 1998;22:759–774.
104. Famularo R, Fenton T, Kinscherff R, Ayoub C, et al. Maternal and child posttraumatic stress disorder in cases of child maltreatment. *Child Abuse & Neglect.* 1994;18:27–36.
105. Malt UF, Hoivik B, Blikra G. Psychosocial consequences of road accidents *European Psychiatry.* 1993;8:227–228.
106. Mayou R, Bryant B, Dunthie R. Psychiatric consequences of road accidents *British Medical Journal.* 1993;307:647–651.
107. Shalev AY, Schreiber S, Galai T, Melmed R. Posttraumatic stress disorder following medical events. *Br. J of Clin Psy.* 1993;32:352–357.
108. Kutz I, Shabtai H, Solomon Z, Neumann M, et al. Posttraumatic stress disorder in myocardial infarction patients: Prevalence study. *Israel J of Psychiatry and Related Science.* 1994;31:48–56.
109. Kessler RC, Sonnega A, Bromet E, et al. Posttraumatic stress disorder in the national comorbidity survey. *Arch Gen Psychiatry.* 1995;52:1048–1060.
110. Fukunishi I, Sasaki K, Chishima Y, Anze M, et al. Emotional disturbances in trauma patients during the rehabilitation phase: Studies of posttraumatic stress disorder and alexithymia. *Gen Hosp Psychiatry.* 1996;18:121–127.
111. Van der Kolk BA. The body keeps the score: memory and the evolving psychobiology of posttraumatic stress. *Harv Rev Psychiatry.* 1994;1:253–265.
112. Van der Kolk BA, McFarlane AC, Waisaeth L, eds. *Traumatic Stress: The Effects of Overwhelming Experience on Mind, Body, and Society.* New York: Guilford; 1996.
113. Yehuda R. Psychoneuroendocrinology of posttraumatic stress disorder. *The Psychiatric Clinics of N. A.* 1998;21:359–379.
114. Schachter CL, Stalker CA, Teram E. Toward sensitive practice: Issues for physical therapists working with survivors of childhood sexual abuse. *Phys Ther.* 1999;79:248–261.
115. Lilienfeld R. *The Rise of Systems Theory.* New York: Wiley; 1978.
116. Capra F. *The Turning Point.* New York: Simon & Schuster; 1982.
117. Capra F. The concept of paradigm and paradigm shift. *Re-Vision.* 1986;9:3.
118. Capra F. *The Web of Life: A New Scientific Understanding of Living Systems.* New York: Anchor Books, Doubleday; 1996.
119. Gorelik G. Principle ideas of Bogdanov's "tektology": The universal science of organization. *General Systems.* 1975;20:3–13.
120. Bertalanffy LV. *General Systems Theory.* New York: Braziller; 1968.
121. Cannon WB. *The Wisdom of the Body.* Rev. ed. New York: Norton; 1939.
122. Weiner N. *Cybernetics.* Cambridge, MA: MIT Press; 1948.
123. Bateson G. *Mind and Nature: A Necessary Unity.* New York: Dutton; 1979.
124. Hoffman L. *Foundations of Family Therapy: A Conceptual Framework for Systems Change.* New York: Basic Books; 1981.
125. Bowen M. *Family Therapy in Clinical Practice.* Northvale, NJ: Jason Aronson; 1978.

126. Kerr ME, Bowen M. *Family Evaluation: The Role of the Family as an Emotional Unit That Governs Individual Behavior and Development*. New York: Norton; 1988.
127. Weinhandle, F. *Gestalthaftes Sehen*. Darmstadt: Wissenschaftliche Buchgelsellschaft; 1960.
128. Kepner J. *Body Process*. New York: Gardner Press; 1987.
129. Odum E. *Fundamentals of Ecology*. Philadelphia: Saunders; 1953.
130. Devall B, Sessions G. *Deep Ecology*. Salt Lake City, UT: Peregrine Smith; 1985.
131. Peak D, Frame M. *Chaos Under Control: The Art and Science of Complexity*. New York: Freeman and Co.; 1994.
132. Prigogine I, Stengers I. *Order out of Chaos; Man's Dialogue with Nature*. Toronto: Bantam Books; 1984.
133. Korr IM. Osteopathic research: the needed paradigm shift. *JAOA*. 1991; 91:156, 161–168,170–171.
134. Sabatino F. Mind and body medicine. A new paradigm? *Hospitals*. 1993;67:66,68,70–72.
135. Wells-Federman CL, Stuart EM, Deckro JP, Mandle CL, et al. The mind-body connection: the psychophysiology of many traditional nursing interventions. *Clin Nurse Spec*. 1995;9(1):59–66.
136. Sommer SJ. Mind-body medicine and holistic approaches. The scientific evidence. *Aust Fam Physician*. 1996;25:1233–1237,1240–1241,1244.
137. Taylor E, Lee CT, Young JD. Bringing mind-body medicine into the mainstream. *Hosp Pract (Off Ed)*. 1997;32:183–184,193–196.
138. Chiarmonte DR. Mind-body therapies for primary care physicians. *Prim Care*. 1997;24:787–807.
139. Grace VM. Mind/body dualism in medicine: The case of chronic pelvic pain without organic pathology: a critical review of the literature. *Int J Health Serv*. 1998;28:127–151.
140. Capra F. *The Tao of Physics: An Exploration of the Parallels Between Modern Physics and Eastern Mysticism*. 3rd ed. Boston: Shambhala; 1991.
141. Wolf FA. *Taking the Quantum Leap: The New Physics for Non-Scientist*. New York: Perennial Library, Harper & Row; 1989.
142. Cohen IB, Whitman A, assisted by Bedenz J. *The Principia: Mathematical Principles of Natural Philosophy/Isaac Newton; a New Translation*. Berkley: University of California Press; 1999.
143. Kaku M, Thompson J. *Beyond Einstein: The Cosmic Quest for the Theory of the Universe*. Rev. ed. New York: Anchor Books, Doubleday; 1995.
144. Bohm D. *Wholeness and the Implicate Order*. New York and London: Routledge; 1980.
145. Herbert N. *Quantum Reality: Beyond the New Physics an Excursion into Metaphysics . . . and the Meaning of Reality*. New York: Anchor Books, Doubleday; 1985.
146. Davies P. *God and the New Physics*. New York: Touchstone Books, Simon & Schuster; 1984.
147. Darling D. *Zen Physics: The Science of Death, the Logic of Reincarnation*. New York: Harper-Collins; 1996.
148. Gleick J. *Chaos: Making a New Science*. New York: Penguin Books; 1987.
149. Goldberger AL, et al. Nonlinear dynamics in heart failure: Implications of long-wavelength cardiopulmonary oscillations. *Am Heart J*. 1984;107:612–615.
150. Goldberger AL, Bhargava V, West BJ. Nonlinear dynamics of the heartbeat. *Physica*. 1985;17D:207–214.
151. Speelman B, Larter R, Worth RM. A coupled ODE lattice model for the simulation of epileptic seizures. *Chaos*. 1999;9:795–804.
152. Larter R, Worth RM, Speelman B. Nonlinear dynamics in biochemical and biophysical systems: From enzyme kinetics to epilepsy. In: Walleczek J, ed. *Self-Organized Biological Dynamics and Nonlinear Control by External Stimuli*. Cambridge, MA: Cambridge University Press; 2000:44–65.
153. Kauffman ES. *The Origins of Order: Self-Organization and Selection in Evolution*. Oxford, England: Oxford University Press; 1993.

3

Historical and Comparative Review of Indirect Methods

Exaggeration Method

Andrew Taylor Still (1828–1917), the founder of osteopathy, advocated and practiced a highly refined and sensitive approach to patient handling and respect for tissues. Little actually is known about the specifics of his manipulative techniques, as he apparently intentionally refrained from writing about them in any detail. However, the specifics of his work are still a topic for discussion in the literature.[1] Still's grandson George Andrew Laughlin, D.O., is thought to have inherited his knowledge and skill base, which later influenced the development and teaching of Functional technique by Edward Stiles, D.O., at Michigan State University. Thus, there is a possible line of connection and continuity from the original osteopathic insight to the present day indirect methodology

Indirect techniques are referred to as the *exaggeration method* in some older references. In *Osteopathic Mechanics*, written in 1915, Ashmore stated:

> There are two methods commonly employed by osteopathists in the correction of lesions, the older of which is the traction method, the later the direct method or thrust. Those who employ the traction method secure the relaxation of the tissues about the articulation by what has been termed exaggeration of the lesion, a motion in the direction of the forcible movement which produced the lesion, as if its purpose were to increase the deformity . . . The exaggeration is held, traction made upon the joint, replacement initiated and then completed by reversal of forces.[2]

In 1949, William G. Sutherland's cranial work was described as an indirect or exaggeration technique with an emphasis on the ligamentous structures. The "point of balanced tension" was sought throughout the manipulative procedure, as awareness of tissue texture changes in response to movement was advocated.[3]

Functional Technique

Indirect manipulative work was further developed and established when Hoover and Bowles began to write about Functional technique.[4-6] Harold Hoover was part of the Academy of Applied Osteopathy's effort to initiate a national program of education in the 1940s.[4] The purpose of this program was to improve postgraduate instruction, ability, and proficiency of practice, "attainable only by those who constantly apply these principles (of Still)."[5] This began the resurgence of indirect osteopathic work, which has continued to the present day.

For comparison, a brief and simplified overview of functional technique is described here. Functional method, which requires a very advanced training and skill base to administer properly, looks at the interrelationship between structure and function, with a functional focus.[7] For example, the vertebra is thought not to be out of place (a structural perspective), but rather it is dysfunctional in relationship to other vertebral segments when movement (function) is introduced into the system. The focus is on restoring quality of movement, regarding ease (not bind) of tissues.

There is a constant interface between diagnosis and treatment with Functional technique. The diagnostic process starts with an initial screening, where signs of asymmetry in structure, tissue, and motion are evaluated.[8] This leads the operator to a local scan of involved areas and finally determination of the specific segmental dysfunction, which represents the area of greatest restriction. Positional diagnosis and other motion tests are repeated after each release to determine the effectiveness of the procedure and guide the operator to the next area of greatest restriction.

The palpating or "listening hand" is key in all indirect functional procedures. The segmental dysfunction is monitored continuously, through palpation, during treatment procedures by the listening hand. The listening hand provides information about response at the level of the segmental dysfunction, as the operator introduces motions into the system with the "motion hand." The palpating hand determines that the state of "dynamic neutral" is maintained throughout the intervention. Bowles originally described dynamic neutral: "Dynamic neutral is a state in which tissues find themselves when the motion of the structure they serve is free, unrestricted and within the range of normal physiological limits."[9] He continued with further clarification:

The term dynamic means that the structure is moving, is a condition of living dynamics; the term neutral means that the action and reaction of the serving tissues stay in normal, or neutral, limits during that motion.[9]

According to Greenman, there are three categories of Functional technique: release by positioning, balance and hold, and dynamic functional procedures.[8] These three procedural methods will be briefly described. The release by positioning method described is Jones's Strain-CounterStrain® system, which will be discussed in the following section.

Balance and hold is described as stacking ranges of movement, then adding the respiratory component by holding an inhalation or exhalation, whichever phase is consistent with more ease in the patient's system. A dynamic process ensues as the operator introduces movements of flexion, extension, side bending, rotation, translation, and then adds the respiratory component during the hold phase of 5–30 seconds. This procedure is repeated from the new balance point until the restriction releases and the range of motion increases.

With the dynamic functional procedures, the listening hand monitors the segmental dysfunction as more varied series of motions are introduced by the motive hand. The operator directs the movement patterns into a path of ease until the dysfunction releases and a normal pattern is restored. This method is thought to "ride out" the dysfunction and restore a normal tracking mechanism at the involved segment.

Jones Strain-CounterStrain

Lawrence Jones, D.O., from Onterio, Oregon (1913–1996), first wrote about his discoveries with indirect work in "Spontaneous Release by Positioning" in 1964.[10] In this article, he described his early successes with positioning as a means to address somatic dysfunction, when his efforts at manipulation were not successful. He continued exploring these concepts in the body of his work, published as *Strain and Counterstrain* in 1981.[11] An updated revised version of this book was published in 1995 as *Jones Strain-CounterStrain.*[12]

Jones helps to clarify his perspective of the underlying difference between Strain-CounterStrain and Functional technique:

Whereas his [Hoover's] dynamic neutral concept sought a bilateral balance of tension fairly near the anatomic neutral position, the concept of the position of spontaneous release focused on the disorder as unilateral and moved to the position of greatest ease of the abnormally tense side, ignoring the well side. This was always at or close to an actual position of strain.[12]

The title of Jones's work is based on his understanding of the underlying physiology of somatic dysfunction. The neuromuscular dysfunction is found not in the muscle that is strained but in the antagonist, or counterstrained, muscle. The counterstrained muscle goes from minimal afferent input into the CNS, during the strain, to registering a very high afferent input just after the strain. The proprioceptors report that the muscle is strained before it even reaches a neutral resting length. This locks the neuromuscular dysfunction in place and the propriceptive misformation continues until the position of initial strain is revisited slowly, with no surprises to the CNS.[12]

Tenderpoints are used by Jones for diagnosis as well as monitoring patient response during treatment. There is significant overlap of these tenderpoints with other points, such as Travell's myofascial trigger points, acupuncture points, and Chapman's reflex points.[8] Each Jones's tenderpoints relates to a specific joint, so that a decrease in point tenderness of a tenderpoint is thought to indicate improved function at that related joint. These points of hypersensitivity to palpation are located throughout the musculoskeletal system. Jones described both anterior and posterior tenderpoints for spinal and other joints. His discovery of anterior tenderpoints is a significant contribution to the treatment of the spine, which previously focused only on posterior involvement. With the Jones method, a multitude of tenderpoints are initially scanned to determine the most restricted area and the treatment sequence.

Jones discussed treating each joint dysfunction in the position of maximum comfort. A position is specifically described in various supine, prone, or sitting positions for each joint dysfunction and associated tenderpoint. These positions recreate the original position of trauma or injury. The correct position of release will be pain free and the point tenderness of the tender point will decrease, when palpated in this position. The position is held for 90 seconds, during which time the tenderpoint is continuously monitored. Jones emphasized a slow return out of the release position back to a neutral position, which is very important to remember. This will assure no surprises to the CNS and no recurrence of trauma from the original position of injury.

Ortho-Bionomy

Ortho-Bionomy® was developed by British osteopath, Arthur Lincoln Pauls (1929–1997). Pauls studied Jones's work as a student, which inspired his treatment method that came to be known as the phased reflex techniques of Ortho-Bionomy. *Ortho-Bionomy* translates generally into "to correct or straighten through the natural laws of life." This method also has come to be known as the *homeopathy of bodywork.*[13] Little is written on Ortho-Bionomy, although the method is still being taught worldwide. Kain's book offers the most descriptive resource available on the subject to date.[14]

Ortho-Bionomy is a form of somatic reeducation that uses comfortable positioning, gentle relaxing movements, and energetic techniques to stimulate the client's self-corrective reflexes in an effort to promote optimal conditions for healing and to restore homeostasis. The reeducation process includes isometric and isotonic exercises as well as postural and other awareness exercises. This respectful, nonforceful approach offers the client possibilities for change while affirming innate body wisdom and knowledge. The approach, taught to lay persons as well as professionals, is relatively easy to learn. The Jones inspired tenderpoints are reduced in number and simplified to a great extent. Although a few muscular releases are described in this method, it is taught primarily from an osteopathic joint perspective, due to Pauls's background. Pauls advocated compression of the joint during the release hold, as a means to decrease the release time from Jones's recommended 90 seconds to 20–30 seconds.

Positional Release Technique

Positional Release is a term used to describe a number of variations of treatment methods that share the commonality of placing patients in positions of comfort and moving the affected tissues away from the restrictive barrier into ease. The goal with all these techniques is to trigger a physiological response to relieve neuromuscular dysfunction.[13] The term *Positional Release* came from Jones's original article, "Spontaneous Release by Positioning."[10]

The first chapter in Chaitow's *Positional Release Techniques* is the most comprehensive comparison of such techniques found in the literature.[13] He discussed Functional technique and Strain-CounterStrain in depth and mentioned other variations of indirect work, including facilitated Positional Release (FPR), induration technique, Goodheart's approach, and Chaitow's integrated neuromuscular inhibition technique.

Stanley Schiowitz, D.O., developed FPR in 1990, which includes aspects of both Functional technique and Strain-CounterStrain.[15,16] He advocated finding the neutral position of the spine in the sagittal plane (regarding flexion and extension) that promotes a decrease in tissue tension and then adds crowding of the tissues or facilitation that includes compression and torsion. This is thought to release the hypertonic tissues in 5 seconds or less. The palpation in FPR is more consistent with Functional technique, which monitors tissue tension not a tenderpoint.

Marsh Morrison described a different palpation approach with induration techniques (1969).[13] He suggested using a very light touch along the paraspinal muscles to determine a "drag" sensation, which relates to increased hydrosis from sympathetic activity, followed by deeper pressure of tissues to confirm involvement. This target area around the transverse process is held with firm thumb pressure while the most adjacent spinous process is taken toward it to create a slack and decreased pain in the involved tissues. Each position is held for 20 seconds and the entire spine can be addressed in this fashion.

George Goodheart, who developed applied kinesiology, suggested a modified and less rigid Jones approach to indirect work.[13] He looks for tenderpoints in the antagonist muscles to the muscles that are actively moving the patient when the restriction or pain is noted. For example, with pain on extension of the spine, the tenderpoints are found in the flexors (psoas muscle) or with painful left neck rotation the tenderpoints are found in the muscles involved with right rotation. Goodheart suggested that a muscle requiring strain-counterstrain will weaken when assessed by using a short isometric contraction. He also uses a neuromuscular stretch technique to the tissues around the dysfunctional muscle spindles during the hold that reduces the hold time to 30 seconds.

Chaitow's integrated neuromuscular inhibition technique (INIT) is a combination of Strain-CounterStrain, muscle energy, and direct inhibition techniques.[13] He advocated positioning a trigger point of a given muscle in a position of ease for 20–30 seconds while administering direct ischemic pressure continuously or intermittently. He followed this release with an isometric contraction of the same muscle just released to obtain an effect of relaxation following the contraction. He finished the treatment sequence with a direct stretch of the hypertonic tissues. An alternative method he suggested following a release is to place the released muscle in a stretched position while having the patient actively contract this target muscle. This latter approach is designed to release contractions and break down fibrotic tissue. Chaitow's INIT techniques appear to be more direct than indirect in nature.

Deig Positional Release Techniques

A less rigid, more dynamic approach to Positional Release is presented in this book. The main emphasis here is to treat what you find, be aware of patient response, and allow that to guide the treatment process. At times, a Jones proprioceptive model of treating the antagonist to the strained muscle is used; at other times, a nociceptive model that targets muscles involved in the withdrawal response. The Positional Release techniques presented in this book include elements from several indirect methods notably Functional technique, Ortho-Bionomy, and Strain-CounterStrain. A brief description is given here, but see Chapter 5 on treatment, Chapter 6 on patient response, and Chapters 7, 12, and 17 on muscular, joint, and isometric application for more detail.

The release positions presented for muscles are based on applied anatomy and the joint releases are based on modified joint mobilization techniques. Involved trigger points are treated but not described as unique to this method. Trigger points can be from Jones,[12] Travell,[17,18] Chapman,[19] acupuncture,[20] or other myofascial or reflex points.[21,22]

The type of palpation advocated includes aspects from both Functional and Strain-CounterStrain methods, depending on the target tissue being addressed. Jones-type[12] tenderpoint monitoring is used for specific myofacial or periosteal trigger points. Palpation more similar to the "dynamic neutral" described in functional methods[7] is used for joint releases and with muscular releases when no specific trigger point is being monitored. This palpation monitors tissue tension more globally on both sides of the joint or throughout the involved muscle or muscles being addressed.

Compression often is used to facilitate the release response; however, there are times when traction is required to recreate original traumatic conditions, other times no longitudinal bias is best. Hold times typically are 60–90 seconds but vary based on palpation of patient response. Positional Release is not a pressure technique. Deeper ischemic pressure can be applied in the release positions described. However, this is thought to be direct work and not part of the release sequence but rather a combination of direct and indirect techniques.

Releases are followed by isometric contractions of the antagonist to the release muscle. Unlike Chaitow's method, which targets the hypertonic muscle (maximal contraction results in maximal relaxation), these isometrics are thought to further decrease the hypertonus of the released muscle through reciprocal inhibition.

The development of the Positional Release technique came out of years of study, clinical practice and experimentation, and collaboration with colleagues. The influences of Ortho-Bionomy techniques,[14] Jones's[12] work, and Functional techniques[7] are evident in this work. However, all these approaches clearly are osteopathic in nature, and this book presents indirect work from a physical therapy perspective with a strong emphasizes on a muscular (anatomical and isometrics) and joint mechanics foundation. The physical therapy profession and our patients may greatly benefit from adding indirect work to their skill base. The following three chapters on examination and evaluation, intervention, and patient response develop the specifics of this indirect physical therapy approach to treatment.

References

1. Van Buskirk RL. A manipulative technique of Andrew Taylor Still as reported by Charles Hazzard, D.O. in 1905. *J Am Osteopath Assoc.* 1996;96:597–602.
2. Ashmore EF. *Osteopathic Mechanics.* Kirksville, MO: Journal Printing Co.; 1915:72.
3. Lippincott HA. The osteopathic technique of Wm. G. Sutherland, D.O, In: Northup TL, ed. *Yearbook of the Academy of Applied Osteopathy.* Ann Arbor, MI: Edwards Bros.;1949:1–24.
4. Hoover HV. The academy program of education. *Yearbook of the Academy of Applied Osteopathy.* Ann Arbor, MI: Cushing-Malloy; 1950:45–46.
5. Hoover HV. Fundamentals of technique. *Yearbook of the Academy of Applied Osteopathy.* Ann Arbor, MI: Edwards Bros;1949:25–41.
6. Bowles CH. A functional orientation for technic. A tentative report on functional approach to specific osteopathic manipulative problems developed in the New England Academy of Applied Osteopathy during 1952–54. *Academy of Applied Osteopathy Yearbook.* Part I, 1955: 177–191; Part II, 1956:107–114; Part III, 1957:53–58.
7. Johnson WL, Friedman HD. *Functional Methods.* Indianapolis: American Academy of Osteopathy; 1994.
8. Greenman PE. *Principles of Manual Medicine.* Baltimore: Williams & Wilkins; 1989.
9. Bowles CH. "Dynamic neutral"—A bridge. Center Harbor, NH: *Yearbook of the Academy of Applied Osteopathy.* 1969:1–2.
10. Jones LH. Spontaneous release by positioning. *D.O.* 1964;4:109–116.
11. Jones LH. *Strain and Counterstrain.* Colorado Springs, CO: American Academy of Osteopathy; 1981.

12. Jones LH, with Kusunose RS, Goering EK. *Jones Strain-CounterStrain.* Boise, ID: Jones Strain-CounterStrain; 1995.
13. Chaitow L. *Positional Release Techniques: Advanced Soft Tissue Techniques.* New York: Churchill Livingstone;1996.
14. Kain K with Berns J. *Ortho-Bionomy®: A Practical Manual.* Berkeley, CA: North Atlantic Books; 1997.
15. Schiowitz S. Facilitated Positional Release. *J Am Osteo Assoc.* 1990;2:145–156.
16. Schiowitz S. Facilitated Positional Release. In: Digiovanna E. *An Osteopathic Approach to Diagnosis and Treatment.* Philadelphia: Lippincott; 1991.
17. Simons DG, Travell JG, Simons LS. *Travell and Simons' Myofascial Pain and Dysfunction: The Trigger Point Manual,* Vol. 1. *Upper Half of Body.* 2nd ed. Philadelphia: Williams & Wilkins; 1999.
18. Travell J, Simons D. *Myofascial Pain and Dysfunction,* Vol 2. Baltimore: Williams & Wilkins; 1992.
19. Owens C. *An Endocrine Interpretation of Chapman's Reflexes; by the Interpreter.* 2nd ed. Indianapolis: American Academy of Osteopathy; 1999.
20. Lu J, Cui Y, Shi R. *Chinese Acupuncture and Moxibustion.* Shanghai: Publishing House of Shanghai College of Traditional Chinese Medicine; 1990.
21. Byers DC. *Better Health with Foot Reflexology: The Original Ingham Method.* St. Petersburg, FL: Ingham Publishing; 1983.
22. Carter M. *Body Reflexology: Healing at Your Fingertips.* West Nyack, NY: Parker Publishing Co.; 1983.

4

Examination and Evaluation

Initial Contact

Evaluation begins the interactive dance between two systems, the therapist and the patient. During the initial contact with a patient, our job is to interview, observe, pinpoint, measure, objectify, determine the course for an action plan, predict time-specific outcomes, and implement treatment—all within an hour or less of evaluation time. Considering the immense complexities of this process and the time constraints we function under, it is no wonder therapists want pat answers to the questions of how to evaluate and where to begin the treatment process. Unfortunately, this book will not provide these answers. The process of evaluation and treatment as an open-ended question, with many avenues or approaches to the goal of successful intervention.

The concept to consider, from a relational systems perspective, is the meeting ground of the two systems are involved. The therapist's worldview, propensities, nature, inclinations, and mind set will determine much about the evaluation process, as this is half of the interactive dance. There is no right or wrong here, just an understanding of who you are and what strengths and weaknesses you bring to the table. Do you function primarily from a strict mechanical model, from an organizational perspective, or do you identify more with the gestalt of the system with which you are interacting? Ideally, you will bring some aspect of each of these as well as other tools of awareness and skill base to the evaluation process.

Each therapist will approach evaluation and treatment in a unique fashion. Since our clinical and personal belief systems shape our reality, then what we observe and interpret during the evaluation process can be influenced by these beliefs. It is important to honor your own ways of making sense of the immense complexity of the dance and allow your own signature approach to develop through time and practice.

Palpation—An Evaluation Tool

Layer palpation is used to examine and evaluate involved tissues, localize the treatment area and help monitor patient response in the target tissues during and after Positional Release intervention. Palpation skill is required to identify the three criteria associated with somatic dysfunction: asymmetry of structure or function, joint motion (hyper- or hypomobile), and tissue texture abnormalities, according to Greenman.[1] He described both static and dynamic palpation. In static palpation, no movement is introduced by the practitioner, as he or she identifies the qualities of the tissues, such as temperature, dryness, moisture, texture, and thickness. In dynamic palpation, both compression and shear movement of the target tissue is evaluated by the introduction of motion. The dynamic palpation process allows for the determination of normal and abnormal range of motion of soft tissues and bony structures in multiple directions. Palpation also increases the awareness of both the patient and the practitioner to detect changes with intervention, determine optimal positioning, and sense quality of movement and ease or bind of tissues.

In *Touching*, Ashley Montagu developed and explored the significance of the skin.[2] He reminded us that the skin arises with the nervous system from the ectoderm or outermost embryonic cell layer. He stated,

> *The central nervous system, which has as a principle function keeping the organism informed of what is going on outside it, develops as the internal portion of the general*

surface of the embryonic body. The rest of the surface covering, after the differentiation of the brain, spinal cord, and all the other parts of the central nervous system, becomes the skin and its derivatives—hair, nails, and teeth. The nervous system is, then, a buried part of the skin, or alternatively the skin may be regarded as an exposed portion of the nervous system.[2]

A layer palpation exercise is recommended before attempting the releases described in this book. Try this simple layer palpation exercise at home, especially if you are learning this material without the benefit of a weekend course. Review of muscular, fascial, vascular, neural, and lymphatic anatomy, in the target area, is advised before proceeding. Although this layer palpation exercise is simple, it requires tremendous concentration; therefore, eliminate outside stimulation and close your eyes, if need be.

The operator is seated comfortably with feet on the floor, spine erect, and forearms supported on the table. The subject is supine for layer palpation of the thigh and seated comfortably or supine for forearm layer palpation. Place both hands with full palmar contact on your partner's forearm or thigh. Begin with static palpation of the skin and subcutaneous fascia to assess tissue texture.

As you work your way down through the layers of soft tissue to the bony structure with dynamic palpation, use light pressure. Remember, less is more, regarding both movement and pressure. Too much movement or pressure interferes with your ability to receive information properly. Pause at target layers or when you need more information and assess with static palpation. Dynamic palpation also can be used at each layer to assess movement bind and ease with directional bias. Explore the skin, subcutaneous fascia, fascial envelope enclosing muscles, muscle fibers (including direction of fibers), musculotendinous junctions, tendons, ligaments, bones, and joint spaces. Vascular pulse and craniosacral rhythm also can be assessed in the target area. From this exercise, determine which tissue layers or bone you would target for intervention.

Area of Greatest Restriction

Indirect methods, such as Functional technique, Strain-CounterStrain®, and Positional Release, vary in their assessment procedures but share the common tenet of treating the most severely involved area first.[3,4] The method of Functional technique taught by Ed Stiles, D.O., identifies dysfunction in the body as originating primarily above or below the diaphragm. From there, further localization of the primary problem is determined through positional diagnosis and assessment or motion restrictions at involved joints. A scan of all questionable areas of involvement determines the area of greatest restriction and treatment sequencing. After each treatment procedure is completed, the scan is repeated. Often secondary restrictions will resolve or clear out after treating the primary restriction. Treatment continues as the next most severe restriction is identified and treated. Treatment sequencing is considered essential to assure effectiveness with the functional method.

Jones's method involves palpation of all tenderpoints to determine which are most tender or where the greatest number of tenderpoints is accumulated.[4] The most involved tenderpoint, which corresponds to the primary area of restriction in the spine, is treated first. Jones advocates treating proximal to distal by first addressing spinal dysfunctions and then the extremities. Until a considerable skill base is reached with this method, evaluation of so many tenderpoints remains a somewhat lengthy prospect.

The Positional Release method described here uses a more functional assessment to determine the target zone and the area of greatest restriction. The target zone can be identified by observing movement and function, determining organizational patterns in the patient's musculoskeletal system, or using other methods of assessment known to the therapist. Once a target zone has been identified, further in-depth examination procedures are used to pinpoint the location of greatest involvement.

Locating the Target Zone

The patient's report about the areas of involvement often is very useful in determining generally where to start treatment. However, this is not entirely reliable; therefore, function rather than pain needs to be your primary focus. To locate the target zone, have the patient verbally identify a motion or function, which he or she finds limiting in daily life. If possible, observe the person performing the activity or function of concern or an approximation of it. If the patient is unable to identify a specific dysfunctional pattern, watch him or her walk, go from sitting to standing and back, from a supine position to sitting and back, roll over, shift weight while standing or sitting—these or similar activities may clue you into the individual's organizational patterns.

During the observation, attempt to determine the area(s) of the body that may be limiting the function in question. If it is still unclear to you, break down the function into simpler movements or units of motor activity and continue to observe until you are able to determine the pattern. Often, the patient organizes all movement around a single area of the body. This area, for example, a shoulder, would engage with all movements and activities. This would be the target zone for further investigation.

Identifying relevant traumatic events through an extensive patient history during the initial evaluation can help focus appropriate intervention through determining the organizational patterns of the individual as well. If a significant trauma has occurred, attempt to recreate the patient's position at the time of the injury. The area of greatest restriction also may be found by examining the involved joints and soft tissues in the region of the body where the vectors of force are thought to have entered their system. See the discussion on force vectors in the Chapter 5 section "Fascial Strain Patterns."

It is important to consider whether the patient's range of motion has been displaced by traumatic impact. The restrictive barrier diagrams (Figures 4-1 and 4-2) may help the

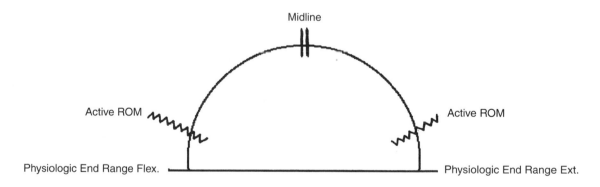

Normal Flexion and Extension Range of Motion Schematic

Figure 4-1: Range of motion for flexion and extension.

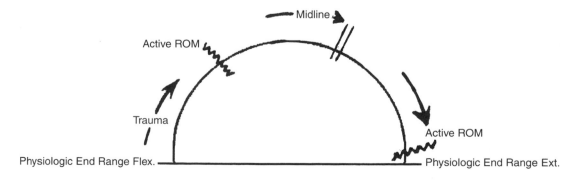

Changes in Flexion and Extension Schematic Due to Trauma

Figure 4-2: The effect of trauma on flexion and extension in range of motion.

practitioner understand how trauma can alter the patient's available range of motion. Figure 4-1 shows active range of motion (AROM), physiological range of motion, and the midline or neutral center of motion in a single plane of motion, under normal conditions. Figure 4-2 shows the effect of trauma, where there is an increase in AROM and shift of midline in the direction of trauma and a decrease of AROM in the direction opposite the trauma.

Treatment with Positional Release involves recreating the original position of injury or taking the patient into the displaced ROM to find the release position. Remember this is a simplified schematic occurring in one plane of motion, when in reality three planes of motion influence the movement pattern you are observing and, therefore, the position during intervention.

In-Depth Examination of the Target Zone

Once the target zone, which requires further evaluation, has been identified, begin your standard examination procedures. These may include objective measures of range of motion, strength, reflex, and sensory testing and perform other special tests specific to the diagnosis and dysfunction being evaluated. Use whatever tests are at your disposal that are significant to your understanding of the problem. Localize the area of greatest restriction by zeroing in further (with a functional or biomechanical model) through assessment of joint motion and palpation of involved muscles. How muscles typically function from either a postural (tonic, Type I) or dynamic (phasic, Type II) perspective is an important consideration during assessment.[5]

When involvement is found, both tonic and dynamic muscles are treated with Positional Release. However, restrictions are found more commonly in tonic muscles due to several factors: a higher number of muscle spindles are present, tone or shortening is increased, and these muscles often are responsible for chronic holding patterns. Examples of tonic muscles of the upper quarter include sternocleidomastoid, scalenes, upper and middle trapezius, levator scapulae, biceps brachii, and pectorals.[6]

Dynamic muscles often present muscle weakness during examination and with exertion.[4] Stretch weakness may make muscles more vulnerable to injury and trauma and often requires the muscle to work harder to function from a mechanically disadvantaged position. Point tenderness and tissue texture abnormalities can be found in dynamic muscles, although the presentation and intervention vary somewhat. The release position may involve less shortening than with a tonic muscle, but let palpation be your guide. Positional Release may improve the patient's ability to strengthen the involved muscle, if pain or somatic dysfunction is interfering with the strengthening process.

The layer palpation exercise will help which tissues need to be targeted during treatment. Determine if the dysfunction is primarily joint or soft tissue in nature through your examination. Although this is a somewhat artificial delineation because all dysfunction includes both joint and soft tissue aspects, however, a dysfunction certainly can be primarily a joint or soft tissue restriction.

Once you have determined the primary restriction and made note of any secondary restrictions, treatment can follow. The plan of care should identify the involved muscles and joints that will be targeted during treatment and the order of treatment based on severity of restrictions found. See Chapters 7 through 11 for muscular releases and Chapters 12 through 16 for joint releases.

Continuous Evaluation-Reevaluation Process

How do you know if you have actually identified the area of greatest restriction? Identify one or two quick tests for function that is most representative of the dysfunctional pattern, such as range of motion or a simple movement. Frequent repetition of this measure will give both the patient and therapist feedback about the progress or lack of response. If range of motion or function is improved in a subjective or objective way, you are on the right tract.

If no change is noted after several attempts, reconsider whether you identified correctly the area of greatest restriction and the target tissues. Assessing the target zone and determining the treatment sequence involves a high level of skill, in Positional Release and other indirect techniques. You will do no harm to the patient if you do not correctly identify the area of greatest restriction, but treatment may take longer and not have as successful an outcome.

After the initial evaluation, it is hard to separate evaluation and treatment, as they become interactive. It is important to reassess joint motion or palpate the muscle that you have treated after each release. This will help guide you through the treatment process. Remember that part of patient education involves an awareness of the dysfunction and the changes made through treatment, which will happen only if you reassess often.

Allow patient response to guide the evaluation and treatment process. If the restriction has decreased but has not cleared entirely, repeat the release process. Further restrictions may be present in a muscle or joint, which require a slightly different release position. If you did not feel comfortable with your release procedure, repeat it with a refinement of technique. If no change is palpated in the tissues, the patient may not be responding to the technique; in which case, this may be time to use isometrics or see if the patient can tolerate another technique.

A Systems Approach to Evaluation

The evaluation methods just discussed and described represent a classic osteopathic perspective, where the emphasis is on treating the most involved area first and sequencing treatment. This is a good place to start, but there are times and exceptions to taking this approach. For example, the area of greatest restriction may be too flared or acute to tolerate any intervention. Sometimes, the accumulative effect of multiple traumas or long-standing compensatory patterns in a patient are so severe that the area of greatest restriction is not readily apparent or assessable. Or, perhaps, the therapist has not yet developed the skill base to effectively determine the area of greatest restriction or simply prefers a more intuitive approach to evaluation and treatment when faced with these or other constraints.

From a dynamic systems perspective, entry into any part of the patient's system, will give you information about the whole system. Treatment of any muscle or joint that is a part of the pattern of dysfunction will provide a link of information into the whole system of dysfunction. From this access point, you may be able to follow the ease of motion in the tissues and locate the center focus of the dysfunction. Often, patients give you useful information about connections and relationships that they experience during the treatment process. Although a certain intuitive function is required for this approach, in certain circumstances, it can be of more value than the classic route of investigation. These would include cases where the involvement does not follow a usual pattern of presentation, tests give conflicting information, facial strain patterns are present that override anatomical considerations, or standard testing procedures cannot be carried out.

Evaluation of certain key areas often is useful in determining involvement elsewhere in the system. Assess areas where muscle fibers run in a transverse direction for involvement, as they are thought to harbor more the traumatic involvement and keep chronic holding patterns ingrained. These would include the pelvic diaphragm (see Figure 8-3), respiratory diaphragm (see Figure 9-1), second rib and thoracic inlet (see Figures 14-5 and 14-6), and the cranial base. Check the upper trapezius insertion, suboccipitals, and the O/A areas for the cranial base (see Figures 10-3C, 10-6, and 16-5).

By checking the respiratory diaphragm involvement, the practitioner can discover relational patterns above or below it. For example, the iliopsoas and quadratus lumborum (see Figures 8-1 and 8-2) needs to be examined in relation to the respiratory diaphragm because of common facial attachments. The scalenes and pectoralis minor (see Figures 10-2 and 9-13) are key muscles to check, when treating above the diaphragm, due to their assessory function in breathing.

A Systems Model: The Stability-Flexibility Continuum

When evaluating a patient, it is important to understand his or her clinical presentation from a more comprehensive systems perspective. This may be helpful in determining the appropriate course of treatment, including when to use Positional Release. For example, consider a continuum with stability on one end and flexibility on the other end. At the stability end, characteristics would include low degrees of freedom of motion and high predictability of movement patterns. At the flexibility end, characteristics such as high degrees of freedom of motion and low predictability of movement patterns would be identified.

If we were comparing joints in the body in this fashion, the hip joint would be toward the stability end and the shoulder joint would be at the flexibility end. Regarding diagnoses, examples of excessive stability would include highly patterned athletes or individuals with repetitive movement disorders, while the flexibility category would include those with conditions such as athetoid cerebral palsy and global ligamentous laxity. See Figures 4-3 and 4-4 for a schematic of the two extremes discussed.

With a highly patterned individual typical of overuse syndromes, using Positional Release to address hypertonic muscles and begin the neuromuscular reorganization process can be beneficial. For example, in an athlete or an office worker, motor dysfunction often develops from the constant repetition of a highly patterned activity. The more time the individual spends repeating a specific movement pattern at the exclusion of activities that challenge the neuromuscular system in different ways, the more likely it is that a dysfunction will occur. The lack of variety of movement typical of an industrial society is thought to be responsible for the chronic facilitation of postural muscles.[7] Positional Release techniques to involved muscles and joints will be helpful in addressing the hypertonicity and unlocking the highly patterned behavior. Movement explorations that break up habitual patterning and improve flexibility, such as with Feldenkrais®, also are useful with this type of dysfunction.[8]

The patient with ligamentous laxity would present the following on evaluation: (1) a high degree of flexibility when measuring range of motion, (2) symptoms that vary greatly from day-to-day, (3) a loss of proprioception, (4) difficulty finding the midline, and (5) a high vulnerability to injury. Depending on the severity of the condition, these patients often develop chronic pain syndromes, even at an early age. Although tone generally would be low, often there will be areas of involvement and restriction with hypertonus in attempts to stabilize, as the muscles attempt to do the work intended for ligaments. These would be the target areas for Positional Release. Evaluation must be constant due to the highly changeable and random patterns that present. The focus of

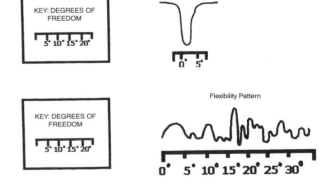

Figure 4-3: Stability pattern, with high predictability of movement.

Figure 4-4: Flexibility pattern, with many possibilities of movement.

rehabilitation is on stability exercises and strengthening but also needs to include Feldenkrais type movement reeducation. This will increase proprioceptive awareness to prevent further injury from excessive end range stress on ligaments and to regain an awareness of midline activity.

Summary of the Examination and Evaluation Process

1. Obtain history of trauma and other relevant events.
2. Observe functional activities.
3. Determine organizational patterns.
4. Locate the target zone.
5. Begin in-depth examination of the target zone.
6. Perform specific tests appropriate to the diagnosis.
7. Assess joint motion.
8. Palpate involved muscles and locate any trigger points.
9. Determine target tissues involved (joint and soft tissue).
10. Determine and perform objective measurement.
11. Determine the area of greatest restriction.
12. Determine and initiate the treatment sequence.
13. Set goals with patient input.
14. Repeat motion tests, palpation, or other objective measurements.
15. Reassess response periodically and modify treatment accordingly.

References

1. Greenman PE. *Principles of Manual Medicine.* Baltimore: Williams & Wilkins; 1989.
2. Montagu A. *Touching: The Human Significance of Skin.* 3rd ed. New York: Perennial Library, Harper & Row; 1986:5.
3. Johnston WL, Friedman HD. *Functional Methods: A Manual for Palpatory Skill Development in Osteopathic Examination and Manipulation of Motor Function.* Indianapolis: American Academy of Osteopathy; 1994.
4. Jones LH, with Kusunose RS, Goering EK. *Jones Strain-CounterStrain.* Boise, ID: Jones Strain-CounterStrain; 1995.
5. Bourdillon JF, Day EA, Bookhout MR. *Spinal Manipulation.* 5th ed. Oxford, England: Butterworth–Heinemann; 1992.
6. Grant R, Janda V. *Physical Therapy of the Cervical and Thoracic Spine: Muscles and Cervicogenic Pain Syndromes.* New York: Churchill Livingstone; 1988.
7. Janda V. Muscles as a pathogenic factor in back pain. In: *The Treatment of Patients,* Proceedings International Federation of Orthopaedic Manipulative Therapists, fourth conference, Christchurch, New Zealand, 1980:1.
8. Bookhout MR. Exercise and somatic dysfunction. *Physical Medicine and Rehabilitation Clinics of North America.* 1996;7:845–862.

5

Intervention and Treatment Considerations

Treatment Procedures Overview

The entire second part of this book describes specific Positional Release techniques that fall into one of three categories: muscular application, joint application, and isometrics. Please see these chapters for more detail regarding treatment procedures, as only a brief overview is presented here. Chapters 7 through 11 address muscular applications, and Chapters 12 through 16 address joint applications. Chapter 17 provides a sample of possibilities for isometrics that follow the releases. Remember that all releases can be followed by an isometric, if necessary, but these are not shown in the book.

The muscular application of indirect principles is through approximation of the origin and insertion. The release positions described are based on anatomical knowledge, but will vary from person to person. The exact position for release needs to be determined though palpation of involved tissues for maximum relaxation. This usually is not maximum shortening, which often triggers an increase in tension in the patient's system, if the position is extreme. Active contraction on the part of the patient during a release does not allow for the necessary afferent reduction.

The joint application procedures are based on joint mobilization assessment with motion testing for bind and ease at the target joint. The motion test determines the preferred direction of motion, which becomes the direction for the release position. Motion is considered in all three planes and stacked to facilitate the release. Anterior-posterior and medial-lateral motion is addressed first, then fine tuning is done by adding the rotation (torsion) component and longitudinal compression or distraction as needed.

The isometrics in this book follow the both muscular and joint releases with a contraction, of the antagonist to the muscle being treated, out of the release position. This is thought to further inhibit the hypertonic muscle that was just released through reciprocal inhibition and to engage the hypotonic muscle on the opposite side of the joint to promote more muscle balance.

Palpation with Indirect Intervention

Development of a high level of skill with palpation is essential for all manual therapy techniques, but this is especially true for indirect work. With all indirect work, palpation actually is a part of the release procedure, rather than something done before and after a technique to assess patient response, as with joint mobilization.[1] Two main palpation models have been described in indirect work: the Strain-CounterStrain®[2] approach to palpation of tenderpoints and the Functional technique,[3] dynamic neutral approach. Variations on both approaches are used with the Positional Release techniques described here. Use the Strain-CounterStrain[2] tenderpoint model of palpation with muscle releases that involve specific trigger points. However, with more global releases of large muscle masses, involvement of several muscles that need to be considered at once or involvement of both sides of a joint, palpation becomes more similar to that described by the Functional method. Here, all the tissues surrounding the joint are in their most relaxed position. This position, where all tensions are equal and minimized, would be consistent with afferent reduction.

Palpation also is used to determine the length of the hold with Positional Release. Generally, releases are held 60–90 seconds; however, at times a longer or shorter hold time is more appropriate, as determined through your palpating hand. In a research project comparing a single session Positional Release or stretch to a control group, there appeared to be a trend toward increased response with an increased hold time of 90 seconds, compared to the 60 seconds with the Positional Release group.[4] A surface electromyogram (EMG) was used as the measure in this study. See Figure 5-1 for a graph of these findings.

Treatment Variations

All the releases described in this book can be adapted to the patient's needs or restrictions or changed at the therapist's discretion with knowledge of anatomy and joint mobilization procedures. The release positions can be modified or created based on considerations such as the size of the patient or therapist and other limitations such as table height or the patient's ability to assume a position. For example, a release for a pregnant woman easily could be modified from supine or prone to side lying.

Learning the necessary palpatory skills and underlying principles is more important than memorizing all the techniques presented. Through development of palpatory skills, you will be able to determine the actual position in which maximum relaxation of the target tissues occurs. The position will vary significantly from person to person. This book is for your learning and reference; however, remember the releases shown are merely guidelines in a dynamic process between therapist and patient.

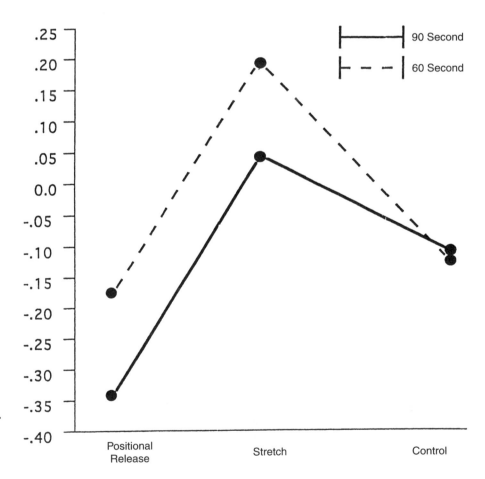

Figure 5-1: The effects of Positional Release on surface EMG activity of the upper trapezius muscles.[2]

Fascial Strain Patterns

During evaluation and treatment, it is important to consider the fascial and connective tissues that are continuous throughout the entire system. The fascial component can account for findings that may not appear to be anatomically correct, from a muscular perspective. Strain patterns often exist, especially after trauma or injury, that extend through groups of muscles, an entire limb or portion of the body, or through the entire body. These fascial strain patterns can be pervasive and may give misleading information to a therapist who functions from a narrow or limited perspective.

Information about an individual's position at the moment of impact and the amount and direction of forces during impact becomes important in treatment, especially if a significant trauma is involved. This information helps identify the direction and extent of force that entered the patient's system. These force vectors provide clues about treatment position and the amount and direction of force that the therapist will need to apply to obtain a release. Keep in mind Newton's third law of motion, for every action there is an equal and opposite reaction.[5] When attempting to initiate a patient response to release trauma from his or her system, it often is necessary to recreate the original position of injury and apply the correct amount of force into the patient's system. As trauma releases, the body can begin to heal and restore function after a significant trauma.

It is important to consider the neuromuscular and skeletal systems as an integrated unit during assessment and treatment. As your palpatory and treatment skills develop, you will begin to observe and treat the strain patterns or force vectors that may be locking the neuromuscular holding patterns in place. Connective tissues are continuous throughout the entire body, connecting muscle to bone, skin to muscle, muscle to organ, viscera to viscera, and therefore all these tissues to each other. Fascial fibers are organized in a multitude of directions, increase in response to stress and trauma, and vary tremendously from person to person; it therefore is impossible to describe specifically what may have occurred with a particular dysfunction in a given individual, except through examination and palpation.

Treatment of fascial restrictions follows the same principles as with other applications described in this book. Determine the bind and ease of involved fascial tissues, follow ease, fine tune, palpate for tissue response, hold the release position until release is complete, and take them slowly out of the release. More than one person may be required to address certain fascial strain problems in patients with multiple areas of involvement.

Integration with Other Techniques

In actual treatment, indirect and direct techniques may be used alternately, based on tissue response, patient acceptance, and the nature and chronicity of the somatic dysfunction. It often is advisable to begin with indirect techniques to gain patients' trust and entry into their nervous systems. It also is important to release any neuromuscular dysfunctions present first, then address the mechanical restrictions that remain with direct work as needed. This softens the tissues and ensures maximum relaxation before doing joint mobilization, muscle energy, or other more direct techniques.

With adaptive shortening of tissues, stretching and deeper direct soft tissue work usually is required to break up adhesions. Extensive fascial involvement and scar tissue also require deeper soft tissue work. Knowledge of release positions is helpful in these cases, as it provides a means to do deeper soft tissue work with increased patient tolerance and acceptance.

Doing Positional Release first to obtain as much resolution of soft tissue and joint restrictions in the involved area as possible is advised. Position the patient in a release position for the target muscle by using pillows, towel rolls, or an assistant, if needed. The point is to keep at least one hand free to do deeper soft tissue work in the release position. The tensor fascia lata and plantar fascia (see Figures 8-6 and 8-15) are examples of releases for muscles with an extensive fascial component, which frequently require deeper soft tissue work.

The deeper soft tissue work can go either with the direction of muscle fibers or across fibers, based on the patient's tolerance and response. Cross fiber work may increase the afferent input and therefore trigger more of a pain response and result in decreased patient tolerance. Static or intermittent deep ischemic pressure in the release position and other suggestions for breaking up adhesions by Chaitow with INIT (integrated neuromuscular inhibition technique) may be beneficial.[6]

Scar release can be done using positioning, by applying the same principles of following ease to release and going into bind with tissues in a position of slack. Both subtle indirect work and deeper direct work can be appropriate, depending on the circumstances. The indirect work is more appropriate for acute or very point tender scars and can be taught as part of self-care activities. Deeper work from positions of tissue ease may be required for more chronic scar formation with adhesions. Again, patient response and compliance should guide your treatment choices.

Releasing soft tissue and joint restrictions prior to stretching activities can be beneficial in increasing range of motion and achieving maximum patient response. Stretching should only be done immediately following a release, if it is tolerated and does not activate a pain response or result in increased tone. Doing a slow sustained stretch in a gentle manner, with the amount of stretch based on the tissue response palpated, will improve results. Gentle movements that challenge the muscle fibers in many directions within a tolerated stretch position also are very effective in increasing range of motion.

The addition of Positional Release to a traditional exercise and rehabilitation program has the advantage of achieving maximum resolution of soft tissue and joint dysfunction in the patient. By normalizing the tone and restoring optimal muscle length, the patient will be more willing and able to meet the demands of reorganization, strengthening, and stretching inherent in a rehabilitation program. Again, Positional Release is recommended to be carried out first, before initiating a strengthening program, and during the strengthening program as needed. The isometric exercises described in this book are a useful way to begin the process of reestablishing normal muscle length and reinforcing new movement patterns.

When establishing an exercise regime for a patient, be aware not to begin too vigorous a program before the pain level has decreased and the structural and functional components have begun to normalize. Until somatic dysfunctions are truly resolved, stress on the system often will result in a return to the dysfunctional pattern. The reorganization process takes time. Work hardening and other vigorous programs can reinforce existing dysfunctional patterns and further irritate the facilitated segment if given too soon or done without first addressing the neuromuscular dysfunction. As discussed previously, the Feldenkrais® method[7,8] of movement reeducation is entirely consistent with the principles of indirect work. With the patient-directed movement exploration characteristic of this method, it is possible to begin the rehabilitation process at a much earlier stage than with a strenuous exercise regime.

Positional Release can be integrated with the treatment of various myofascial trigger points,[9,10] acupuncture[11] or acupressure[12] points, Chapman's points,[13] and other reflex points.[14,15] With these releases, it sometimes is useful to perceive the reflex or trigger point as at the center of a concavity. Positioning the involved soft tissue or body part around the trigger or reflex point you are releasing usually results in a softening effect and release of the involved tissues.

Both therapist and patient will find integrating visualization into the treatment process useful. Visualization of the specific muscle being released will increase the concentration of the therapist, help to pinpoint details such as direction of fibers, and illuminate relationships with other anatomical structures. At times, it also may be beneficial for the patient to have an image of the target muscle or joint being released. The anatomy drawings in this book will be helpful in this aspect of patient education. This will increase patient participation in the release process and often facilitates results. During certain isometrics it is helpful for the patient to visualize the contraction as originating from a certain region, under the direction of the therapist.

Home Program and Self-Treatment

Often a patient has a long-standing, chronic involvement and specific releases are beneficial, but the results do not maintain between treatment sessions. In this case, it is useful to teach a family member to do the release(s) on a daily or more frequent basis than in therapy sessions. Many of the releases shown in this book are appropriate to teach a family member or friend. Generally, the muscular releases and isometrics are easier to teach an inexperienced support person than the joint releases.

Demonstrate to the designated support person two or three specific techniques that you would like to be carried out as a part of a home program. Most laypersons will find the anatomical descriptions interesting, but this may or may not benefit their understanding of the release process. It may be of help to a layperson to describe the area you are targeting for release as the center of a concavity. Teach them to position the body around the target point or tissues to achieve slack or softening there. Have the support person practice in front of you with feedback provided by both patient and therapist.

A few of the techniques presented in this book are appropriate for self-treatment, but with most, it is difficult to achieve the complete relaxation necessary to decrease afferent input into the patient's system. Generally, the patient will need to stay in the position for 5–20 minutes, unless he or she somehow can recreate the approximation of origin and insertion without increasing tension elsewhere in the system.

The iliopsoas releases (see Figure 8-1) can be modified by having the patient lie on the floor with the legs flexed on a couch or large chair, with pillows for support in the release position. The patient can be instructed to do self-palpation to determine if he or she is getting the same results achieved with the therapist in the clinic. The prone quadratus lumborum release (see Figure 8-2B) also is useful for self-care but should be followed by stretching or movement work, especially if a patient reports this as a sleeping position. Staying in a self-release position for more than 20 minutes is not advisable, as it may be counterproductive by creating habitual restriction of already shortened tissues.

Patients can successfully carry out certain releases on themselves, if they are able to achieve complete relaxation, with no active contraction of the involved area. For example, the patella releases can be done as a self-release by having the patient in a long sitting position with the back supported against a wall. From this position, the patient should have two free hands to work on the patellae as described in Figure 13-12. This frequently is given as part of self-care following knee surgery.

Certain foot and ankle releases (see Figures 13-2 through 13-4) can be done similarly, if the patient has adequate range of motion to access the involved foot. Have the patient support him- or herself in a chair, or with long sitting, with one leg flexed at the knee and hip with hip external rotation (Taylor sitting). The involved leg can be supported on pillows, if necessary.

Wrist, finger and forearm releases could also be carried out by supporting the involved arm on a table or knee, while doing the releases with the other hand. Many of the other releases are difficult to do without active contraction on the part of the patient.

References

1. Greenman PE. *Principles of Manual Medicine*. Baltimore: Williams & Wilkins; 1989.
2. Jones LH with Kusunose RS, Goering EK. *Jones Strain-CounterStrain*. Boise, ID: Jones Strain-CounterStrain; 1995.
3. Johnson WL, Friedman HD. *Functional Methods*. Indianapolis: American Academy of Osteopathy; 1994.
4. Deig DK. *The Effects of Positional Release and Stretching on Surface EMG Activity of Upper Trapezius Muscles* [masters thesis]. Indianapolis: University of Indianapolis; 1994.
5. Cohen IB, Whitman A, assisted by Bedenz J. *The Principia: Mathematical Principles of Natural Philosophy/Isaac Newton; a New Translation*. Berkley: University of California Press; 1999.
6. Chaitow L. *Positional Release Techniques: Advanced Soft Tissue Techniques*. New York: Churchill Livingstone; 1996:12–13.
7. Feldenkrais, M. *Awareness Through Movement: Health Exercises for Personal Growth*. New York: Harper & Row; 1972.

8. Rywerant Y. *The Feldenkrais Method: Teaching by Handling.* New Canaan, CT: Keats Publishing; 1983.

9. Travell J, Simons D *Myofascial pain and dysfunction,* Vol 1. Baltimore: Williams & Wilkins; 1983.

10. Travell J, Simons D *Myofascial pain and dysfunction,* Vol 2. Baltimore: Williams & Wilkins; 1992.

11. Lu J, Cui Y, Shi R. *Chinese Acupuncture and Moxibustion.* Shanghai: Publishing House of Shanghai College of Traditional Chinese Medicine; 1990.

12. Houston FM. *The Healing Benefits of Acupressure; Acupuncture without Needles.* New Canaan, CT: Keats Publishing; 1974.

13. Owens C. *An Endocrine Interpretation of Chapman's Reflexes;* by the Interpreter. 2nd ed. Indianapolis: American Academy of Osteopathy; 1999.

14. Byers DC. *Better Health with Foot Reflexology: The Original Ingham Method.* St. Petersburg, FL: Ingham Publishing; 1983.

15. Carter M. *Body Reflexology: Healing at Your Fingertips.* West Nyack, NY: Parker Publishing Co.; 1983.

6

Patient Participation and Response

Patient Participation

To effect an afferent reduction during a release, the patient must be passive in terms of having no active contraction of the treatment area. This has led some to conclude that Positional Release is entirely a passive process on the part of the patient, which is not accurate. Patient responsibility is emphasized as essential to the therapeutic process with Positional Release. The therapist can increase participation by actively engaging the patient during the treatment process in several ways.

Awareness techniques can be used during treatment to increase participation by patient and increase his or her knowledge about the somatic dysfunction. This provides information about changes occurring with treatment for both patient and practitioner. Visualization by the patient, pausing after a release to get patient feedback, and asking the patient to focus in other ways on the area being treated are useful in increasing patient awareness. Discussing the involved muscle that is being released and showing the patient a muscle drawing prior to working on it will improve the ability to visualize the area during treatment. Asking the patient to imagine the muscle softening, lengthening, or letting go often is helpful. Taking a pause during treatment to ask the patient to feel the differences and verbalize the changes felt between two limbs or two sides of the body is of great benefit in increasing awareness after working on an area.

Asking the patient to be still and to focus inside on the treatment area sometimes is required, if a patient engages too much in conversation or social interaction with the therapist. Excessive chatter from the patient sometimes is a defense mechanism, used unconsciously to block the perception of what is really going on in his or her system. This is especially true with a strong emotional overlay, such as anger or sadness after an accident, injury, or abuse. Suggestions to take their breath into the area of involvement or to allow the tissues to soften by making a space for your palpating hand or fingers actively engages the patient in the treatment process, which facilitates results and helps break up patient holding patterns.

Jones suggested getting feedback from the patient when palpating the painful tenderpoint by asking if it is better, worse, or the same after placing the patient in the release position.[1] This increases patient participation and is especially useful when a therapist first starts to use indirect methods and has not fully developed palpation skills or trust in what he or she feels. If a very painful trigger point improves drastically by placing the patient into a release position, the patient often states that you moved your finger even if you kept it in stationary contact the whole time. Getting patient feedback in this way helps keep that person focused on the treatment process and often confirms palpation findings. At times, the patient will provide feedback that is contrary to what is palpated.

Isometric exercises are an excellent means of engaging the patient actively in the release process. By giving very specific tactile and verbal cues, the therapist can obtain an isometric contraction, which recruits the exact fibers needed to correct the somatic dysfunction and realign structural faults. This more precise use of isometric contraction may take several attempts by the patient or the therapist to obtain the desired results. Using more isometrics during a treatment session is recommended to increase patient participation, especially if he or she has difficulty focusing on the treatment process or does not understand what you are trying to accomplish.

Potentiality of Response from a Systems Perspective

From a systems perspective, patient worldview and response are the primary determinants in evaluation and treatment. During evaluation and treatment, the therapist enters the patient's worldview in an effort to effect change in the direction of decreased symptoms and increased function. Therefore, the therapist must be aware of multiple aspects of the patient's worldview and the potentiality of patient response. In addition to the patient's physical aspects of disease or dysfunction, his or her mental, emotional, social and spiritual worldview, and well-being must be taken into consideration. Consider how each of these aspects, especially the emotional context, may effect the therapeutic relationship and intervention.

Mental blockages to progress in therapy often involve secondary gains that, consciously or unconsciously, keep the patient in a dysfunctional state. This may relate to getting attention or special treatment from significant others as a result of continuing in a pattern of dysfunction. Unfortunately, mental blocks to recovery sometimes are involved when legal or financial gains can be made following an accident or injury. Awareness of this possibility may influence the therapist's decision about the treatment focus, length of treatment, and possible outside referral, if progress has reached a plateau. It is recommended to increase patient participation in treatment, objectify compliance with a home program, and if appropriate, discuss the patient's motivation or lack thereof in recovery to address these problems. Outside referral to a psychologist, biofeedback therapist, or vocational rehabilitation counselor also may be appropriate.

With consideration of the mind-body paradigm literature reviewed in Chapter 2, it is probably impossible actually to separate the interrelationship between a patient's emotional and physical aspects of dysfunction or assign causation to one set of considerations. However, the strict yet artificial boundaries between a patient's physical and psychological health care, the lack of therapists trained in integrated mind-body methodology, and the professional disinclination regarding cross-disciplinary approaches perpetuate the mind-body split.

In *Job's Body*,[2] Deane Juhan illuminated a more accurate view of body-mind reality:

> *The relationships between our experiences, our feelings, and our body chemistry are undoubtedly far more intricate than we can presently imagine. We have seen how specific mental states effect specific glandular secretions, circulatory patterns, organ functions. If we now remind ourselves that every nerve cell is itself a type of gland, a gland whose chemical secretions are the mechanisms for carrying action potentials from cell to cell, we can appreciate the fact that there is probably no limit to the influencing of function and behavior by feelings and attitudes.*[2]

Physical therapists often elicit an emotional response to treatment when they are seeking to affect only a person's physical well-being. This is especially true when using Positional Release and other techniques that address the central nervous system from an integrated perspective. Emotional responses channeled through the limbic system occur more rapidly than thinking responses processed through the neocortex.[3] Autonomic nervous system "fight or flight" responses can be triggered in a matter of a second through a multitude of sensory stimuli (somatic, visual, tactile, auditory, olfactory) with any emotional overlay.[3]

Memories of both psychological and physical trauma appear to be held almost indefinitely in a patient's system and sometimes are triggered by a certain touch, hold position, or movement. Frequently a patient who reported absolutely no trauma on initial evaluation relate a traumatic incident to the therapist that had occurred many years ago and had been forgotten consciously yet still appears to reside in their unconscious.

The concepts of sensory and traumatic engrams developed by Deane Juhan in *Job's Body* may be helpful in understanding the release of traumatic memories in response to tissue manipulation.[2] He developed the idea of sensory engrams, or templates of sensory records associated with movements, as part of our motor learning process. He credited this sensory memory for control, learning, and repetition of motor skills and sees the muscles as responding to engram information coming through the direct corticospinal and multineuronal pathways in the spinal cord. Engrams are established through life experience and create organizing factors unique to an individual.

The more primitive reflexes of the spinal cord and brain stem may be at odds with the consciously developed patterns of engram response, and therefore antagonist conflicts can occur between mental and physical responses. A life history of emotional or physical trauma can condition a heightened response by association to certain movement patterns, positions, or other triggers, which may not always seem significant to an outside observer or unknowing therapist.

The therapist's observation of body posture, organization, and emotional anatomy can provide some clues as to holding patterns that may represent a patient's emotional or energetic expression or problem areas. Stanley Keleman's *Emotional Anatomy: The Structure of Experience*[4] and Bonnie Bainbridge Cohen's *Sensing, Feeling, and Action: The Experiential Anatomy of Body-Mind Centering*[5] lend considerable insight into this observational skill development. Consider how exposure to repeated traumatic events, such as withdrawal from painful blows, may become locked in a person's system and ultimately reflect in a posture of severe withdrawal or defeat and a heightened response to manipulation of the area that received the blows.

Richard Erskine described the physiological formation of "body scripts" in response to threatening situations, sometimes at a very early age, which continue to influence and condition the individual in negative ways. He stated that, "the scripting process takes place within the tissue of the body as a survival reaction."[6] Left untreated, these scripts can become the cause of many physical illnesses. He recommended that, "Script cure at the physiological level is letting go of the tensions, body armoring, and internal restrictions that inhibit the person from living life fully and easily within his or her own body."[6]

Emotional release can take many forms, including silent or screaming tears, anger, rage or actual reenactment of traumatic events. Attempting to inhibit a response once it is triggered can interfere with their healing process and counter the positive effect of treatment. However, it is very important to ascertain your level of expertise and comfort level when faced with this situation. Emotional releases usually are sudden, unexpected, and without much of a warning, see Chapter 24, "Case Study: Cervical Whiplash Injury."

The immediate need of the patient is for support. Support may be sitting silently, handing the patient a tissue, or just listening to his or her story. Sometimes, no further intervention is necessary. Remember that, unless you are a trained mental health worker, the patient will not expect you to possess expertise in the field of psychology. Know your bounds of practice and, if needed, refer the patient to a trained psychiatrist, psychologist, or social worker for care. Consultation or concurrent treatment with a mental health professional is useful in cases of deeper body-mind trauma or dysfunction or recurrent emotional release episodes during physical therapy, which repeat without any sign of progress.

The social aspects of treatment include consideration about the patient's home life, vocational status, relational propensities or problems, and substance abuse issues. If, for example, the chronic pain or physical dysfunction interferes with the patient's ability to earn a living or is a potential financial threat to the individual's well-being, his or her response to treatment and your direction of treatment will be affected. Issues of will and motivation to recovery often will be influenced by repercussions or rewards in the social arena. Awareness of the bigger picture of the patient's life and the role the physical dysfunction plays is important when considering the course of treatment, treatment response, and discharge plans. Referral to outside professionals such as a psychologist, vocational rehabilitation specialist, social worker, or other health care providers sometimes is the recommended course of action.

Spiritual considerations of treatment that are potentially vast will be simplified for the purposes of this book. Remember that the patient's belief system may be the most powerful operative toward healing in the treatment process. To the best of your ability try to encourage and support the positive implications of beliefs, without judgment, in whatever form they may appear. Otherwise, it is important to remain as neutral as possible, make no assumptions, and above all do not impose your belief system on the patient. If there appears to be a strong spiritual component or blockage to treatment, outside referral to a priest, minister, rabbi, or other spiritual advisor is recommended.

Patient Response with Positional Release

It is important to consider the release response, not only from a theoretical perspective, but also from the perspective of both therapist and patient. Observation of the patient release response, by the therapist, primarily involves gathering data through palpation. The therapist usually will feel a decrease in tension or tone in the involved area once the patient is in the release position. This softening or melting of tissues is the most usual response observed by the therapist, as it indicates successful positioning and a decrease in afferent input into the system. This response is easier to palpate with certain muscles such as the hip adductors (see Figure 8-7B) than with a muscle that requires layer palpation such as the psoas release (see Figure 8-1B).

Other indications of release are observation of a therapeutic pulse during the release and increased warmth or circulation to the area following the release.[7] The therapeutic pulse can be quite strong and fast during the release. It generally does not match the patient's actual vascular pulse rate and its disappearance usually indicates the release is complete.

From the patients' perspective, the release response is more complex, being an interior experience that relates to all aspects of their system, as previously discussed. Patients usually report a feeling of comfort and sometimes relief when placed in an appropriate release position. They may or may not experience the changes in tone or circulation but often report an immediate change in pain level in response to palpation during and following a release. The painful trigger or joint motion may or may not be completely resolved, but usually be some change is reported when asked by the therapist, which helps guide the treatment process.

The possibilities are almost limitless when discussing patient experience. The patient may relate information about sensations or pain in areas distant to that being treated. The release position may trigger an emotional response or awaken a somatic-based memory of trauma or injury. The patient may not report experiencing much change during a treatment session but return to the next visit with a report of increased awareness in some aspect of his or her being. The patient may experience an increase freedom of motion and wish to test this by repeating a challenging movement or function immediately after a treatment session. Occasionally, this will trigger a reoccurrence of spasm or pain, if done too vigorously or too soon, and require you to warn the patient to take it easy immediately following the session or for the rest of the day. The patient simply may not respond to this indirect type of treatment and require a different treatment focus. Consider all possibilities and make your best professional judgment regarding the optimal patient care.

Homeopathic Body Work

Indirect methods, such as Positional Release, are considered by some to be homeopathic in nature. Homeopathic medicine (which literally translates as "same pathos") uses submolecular dosages of natural substances to stimulate the innate healing process of the body.[8–10] Homeopathic treatment is thought to treat the cause of the disease, as compared to most allopathic medicine, which usually focuses on symptomatic treatment of the disease. Frequently, with homeopathic treatment, the symptoms actually become more aggravated or increased during a certain phase of treatment. This, usually referred to as a *healing crisis*, often represents an unstable phase before the reestablishment of a new homeostasis within the patient's system. Figure 6-1 shows an unstable pattern in response to a therapeutic intervention between two stable patterns regarding degrees of freedom of motion. The new pattern is less rigid, with more movement possibilities available than the old holding pattern. In homeopathic medicine, the healing crisis is thought to be a positive signal that the remedy being given is correct and the patient is responding to that remedy.

There are similarities between indirect work and traditional homeopathy, which may account for the observation of a healing crisis or period of exacerbation of symptoms at some point during the treatment process. Recreating the original position of trauma or injury could be seen as an example of "same pathos," being the stimulation for the patient to respond with a self-corrective reflex. Indirect work may address the fundamental cause of the somatic dysfunction more than traditional physical therapy treatments, which provide only symptomatic relief, such as hot packs, ice, or ultrasound, and therefore can be thought of as allopathic in nature.

A healing crisis is more likely to occur with certain patient profiles and during certain times in the treatment process. A patient who has sustained a major impact injury, has had multiple traumas, or has multiple areas of involvement will likely go through a more drastic reorganization of the system, or a healing crisis, before resolution of their symptoms occur. A healing crisis is likely to follow a treatment session in which you have been successful in truly recreating the complex combination of release postures and input of forces necessary to mimic those the patient originally sustained during the trauma. Oftentimes a healing crisis will occur toward the end of treatment, just prior to complete resolution of the symptoms.

When using indirect methods, the patient must be educated about this aspect of treatment, especially if he or she presents severe involvement. During the initial phase of treatment, inform the patient that this kind of therapy is process oriented and determine if he or she is willing to go through that process at this time. Symptoms often change in nature and location, especially during the initial phase of treatment. The patient also may experience muscular soreness, as though having gone through a workout, rather than the pain initially presented. Seemingly, new areas of pain or dysfunction may appear as you peel away the onionskin layers of symptoms. If you perceive a significant response during treatment, it may be a good time to inform the patient of

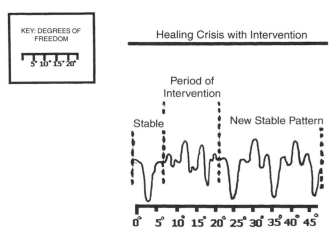

Figure 6-1: Schematic of a healing crisis.

the potentiality of a healing crisis. Suggest that the patient use heat, ice, antiinflammatory medication, or other symptomatic relief, as necessary, following treatment. If the problem or dysfunction is more acute or simple in nature, it may be unnecessary to discuss the healing crisis at all.

Also consider the healing crisis from the perspective of dynamical systems theory, as discussed in Chapter 2. The healing crisis probably represents an unstable phase between two stable phases or a period of pattern disruption. The understanding here is that the unstable phases do not represent equilibrium and therefore will not become an attractor, hence it is temporary. Also remember that the new attractor or pattern most probably will be more functional than the pattern initially presented.

Assess your own willingness and ability to undergo this process with a patient. Keep in mind your options to refer the patient to a more highly skilled therapist or osteopath if you are uncomfortable with your skill base or the patient's level of involvement. You always can choose to treat a patient with another method, which focuses on only relief of symptoms.

References

1. Jones LH, with Kusunose RS, Goering EK. *Jones Strain-CounterStrain.* Boise, ID: Jones Strain-CounterStrain; 1995.
2. Juhan D. *Job's Body: A Handbook for Bodywork.* Barrytown, NY: Station Hill Press; 1987.
3. Goleman D. *Emotional Intelligence.* New York: Bantam Books; 1995.
4. Keleman S. *Emotional Anatomy: The Structure of Experience.* Berkeley, CA: Center Press; 1985.
5. Cohen BB. *Sensing, Feeling, and Action: The Experiential Anatomy of Body-Mind Centering.* Northampton, MA: Contact Editions; 1993.
6. Erskine RG. *Theories and Methods of an Integrative Transactional Analysis.* San Francisco: TA Press; 1997.
7. Rathburn J, Macnab I. Microvascular pattern at the rotator cuff. *Bone and Joint Surgery.* 1970;52:540–553.
8. Boericke W. *Homeopathic Materia Medica: Comprising the Characteristic and Guiding Symptoms of All Remedies.* 9th ed., export ed. New Delhi, India: B Jain Publishers; 1981.
9. Wheeler CE. *An Introduction to the Principles and Practice of Homeopathy.* 3rd ed. Devon, England: Health Science Press; 1948.
10. McCabe V. *Let Like Cure Like; The Definitive Guide to the Healing Power of Homeopathy.* New York: St. Martin's Press; 1997.

Part II

Positional Release Techniques

7

Introduction to Muscular Application

The Muscle Matrix and Its Motor Units

Anatomical descriptions are useful for reducing the enormously complex muscular matrix into manageable functional units for learning and consideration. Although anatomy is highly emphasized in this book, please do not let this limit your capacity to embrace the larger picture of patient presentation. In addition to being a learning aid, the main purpose of the muscular drawings in this book is to help the reader gain a three-dimensional, working perspective of a patient's musculoskeletal system. There is considerable variation of muscle organization and even more variation of the fascial organization from person to person found on dissection. Chronic holding patterns will not be limited to a single muscle but rather involve muscle fibers and motor units from several muscles that need to be addressed in treatment.

Many examples are presented throughout the body of extensive interdigitations of fibers from several muscles, such as serratus anterior, external obliques, and latissimus dorsi fibers on the lateral chest wall below the axilla. In these areas, it often is difficult to identify the exact fibers belonging to one muscle or the other, and treatment therefore should consider all involved muscle fibers and motor units. In *Job's Body*, Deane Juhan best described this integrated concept of muscular organization.[1]

> *So we will be closer to the complex truth in our conceptualization of muscular activity if we regard the body as having only one muscle, whose millions of fiber-like cells are distributed throughout the fascial network and are oriented in innumerable directions, creating innumerable lines of pull. This single muscle may then contract or lengthen any number of fibers distributed in any number of compartments in order to change its consistency and shape in an almost amoeba-like fashion.*[1]

While conceptualizing these dynamics of a muscular system functioning as one global matrix, it is also important to consider intervention from a more local perspective by treating the involved or dysfunctional motor units. Therefore, for the purposes of treatment, consider individual motor units, rather than the whole muscle, and focus on treating the involved motor units, rather than the entire neuromuscular mechanism.

The trapezius muscle is a good illustration of how different parts of a muscle function as individual motor units. The entire muscle is innervated by the spinal accessory nerve and C_3 and C_4 nerve roots, yet there is a large variation of function depending on which fibers or part of the muscle fires. The entire muscle acting together retracts the scapula, however the upper trapezius when acting unilaterally side bends toward and rotates the head away, while the lower trapezius acting alone, draws the scapula in an inferior and medial direction.[2] This ability of motor units to fire independent of one another illustrates the isolated function of motor units within a given muscle and needs to be considered during treatment. Involvement can be isolated to a few motor units, be more global throughout the entire muscle, or extend to several muscles.

Variation in Muscular Releases

The Positional Release technique presented in this book allow for a great deal of flexibility of application. Releases can be done in a wide range of treatment possibilities, from a quite specific application to a more general application, based on your findings, treatment objectives, and patient response. Palpation for a smaller area of treatment focus, such as with a trigger point release, will be more similar to the tenderpoint palpation described by Jones.[3] More general releases may require palpation with broader surface contact to monitor the tissue relaxation response in a larger muscle mass or several target muscles at once.

Releases can be adapted to address very specific restrictions found in the soft tissues. Through refinement of palpation and treatment skill it is possible to zero in on a wide array of tissue texture abnormalities. Multiple areas of involvement in a certain muscle may require several releases to the same muscle, in slightly different release positions, to address all involved motor units. Fine-tuning the basic release positions enables you to address very specific muscular fiber tension patterns. Remember that palpation and patient feedback will be your guide through this process.

A more general release of one or more muscles may be appropriate given your treatment focus or intention. An intermuscular release can be done between two or more muscles, such as with the quadriceps, vastus medialis, lateralis, intermedius, and the rectus femoris (see Figure 8-9C). A midmuscle release can be done with any of the long muscles or groups of muscles, such as with the superficial paraspinals (see Figure 11-1C), by targeting the involved fibers during the release procedure. General releases are useful when attempting to recreate their unique structural patterns, such as with a scoliosis or other prevalent patterns that bias structural alignment.

Nearly all the releases can be modified to suit the needs of both patient and therapist. This book suggests basic release positions based on ease of patient handling and consideration of therapist's body mechanics. Frequently, release options are given in more than one position. Patient and therapist size, patient response, body contours, availability of adjustable table height, and special considerations such as tolerance for positions based the patient's pathology or physiological conditions need to be considered when determining the ideal release position for you and your patients.

Good body mechanics by the therapist are very important. Use your arms to the best mechanical advantage by leaning back with your entire body, with arms extended, to hold a release. This will be more effective than attempting to push up a body part. Remember that a 60- to 90-second hold will be most difficult if you start from an awkward or uncomfortable position. Your discomfort will translate into the patient's system and decrease the probability of success. It is also important to line yourself up with the specific fibers of the muscle that you are releasing to maximize results.

Assessment of Muscular Involvement

Palpatory skill development is the key to accurate assessment of muscular involvement. Review and practice the layer palpation exercise in Chapter 4 to improve your skill base. Palpate the target muscle in a neutral resting position, before taking the patient into a release position. This will provide you baseline information regarding the extent of point tenderness and tissue texture abnormalities before intervening with a release procedure. It is best to repeat palpation of the involved tissue after the release, again from a neutral resting position, to ascertain the effects of the release. Palpation also is used during the release to provide continuous feedback and ensure optimal effectiveness of treatment.

Keep in mind that your palpation pressure needs to be consistent before, during, and after the release. When possible, keep your palpating hand in contact throughout the whole release procedure. This is desirable to assure a high level of accuracy of assessment and reassessment and to increase patient awareness of changes that may have occurred from the release. If the pain has disappeared, the patient often will state that you have moved your palpating hand rather that realize that there has been a change in their response to pressure.

Pressure is used for assessment of point tenderness, but not during the release. Remember less is more regarding palpation pressure. Too much pressure interferes with your ability to perform an accurate assessment. Palpation pressure generally is lighter than the typical physical therapist is used to using when assessing soft tissue restrictions. Tension in the therapist's hands or system again translates into the patient's field and interferes with optimal treatment. The actual amount of pressure used will vary, depending on the body type of the patient, the area being assessed, and the therapist's skill level. Try to be consistent with palpation pressure before and after each release. Remember that Positional Release is not a pressure technique.

When assessing an area for soft tissue restrictions it is important to attempt to keep in mind several informational levels at once. Which specific tissue should be my treatment focus: muscle, fascia, ligament, tendon, or bony attachment? This question often can be addressed through layer palpation. Which groups of muscles are involved? What part of the target muscle is most restricted? How does this restriction relate to the pathology? What is the relationship between this restriction and other parts of the patient's body? What are the relationships to mental, emotional, or other considerations within his or her system? What is the relational aspect between the treating therapist's system and the patient's system? Having a multilevel focus and being able to gather information from a macrocosmic to a microcosmic perspective is of great value when using Positional Release or other treatment procedures. If you can feel other restrictions or significant relationships during the release process, the patient's unique patterns will come alive for you and treatment will become much more effective.

Procedural Considerations During the Release

To effect a decrease in the afferent input, it is important to keep in mind several factors during the release process. Remember that the release procedure needs to be passive, as active contraction on the part of the patient will negate the desired neurological change. If a patient begins to contract the area being released it is advisable to return to a neutral resting position and start again. Go more slowly into the release and do not take the patient into such an extreme position; you may be setting off antagonistic muscles or taking the muscles into a painful range of motion.

The therapist also must provide as much support as possible to the involved area or body parts during the release and coming out of the release. This is why instructions for many releases suggest using the therapist's leg or arm as a support. The use of pillows is recommended as an option if the therapist feels uncomfortable or compromised in any way during the release. Only through adequate support will a patient be able to relax enough to effect a change during a release.

Fine-tuning the position of release can be done through the more gross aspect of positioning or with much more subtle changes through the rotational component, slight variations in your hand placement, or pressure changes that you enter into their system. Through palpatory skill, you will be able to ascertain the ideal position for release, as movement in either direction will slightly increase the tone and tension in the area. This has been compared to finding a station on the radio dial, the reception is best at a certain spot and the signal begins to fade in either direction from the optimal one. For more subtle fine-tuning remember to add the rotational component and longitudinal compression or distraction based on tissue response. Subtle changes in your hand placement or pressure input to release specific target tissues can make a tremendous difference between success or failure with this technique.

Going slowly into and out of the release position is very important for different reasons. Taking the patient slowly into the release position will assure that you do not go past the optimal release position. Taking the patient slowly out of the release position will assure that the original mechanism of injury that began the dysfunction is not repeated. Jones emphasizes the importance of this in *Strain-CounterStrain*®.[3]

Breath can be an important tool to facilitate the release process. Using the patient's breathing to go into the release position is helpful, especially when releasing muscles in the thorax or pelvis or the specific muscles used for breathing such as the diaphragm, scalenes, or pectoralis minor. Ask the patient to take a deep breath in and exhale slowly. Follow the breath and take the patient into the release on the exhalation. Giving cues for patients to relax with each breath or release all the tension in their system on the exhalation is helpful at times. A verbal command to "relax" sometimes can trigger more of a tension response from patients in a lot of pain. This is when focus on their breathing can be very useful in getting a relaxation response. It also may be helpful to ask patients to "let me have the weight of your leg" or use similar verbal cues.

The releases presented in this book generally are taught as static position and hold releases. However, this is just the starting point. If you are engaged in the release process and can perceive the patient's response, the process is dynamic and will take its own course to completion. For example, a release may occur and lead you into one or more successive releases of the same region in a slightly different position, or a relational association (of trauma or dysfunction) to another area of the body may become apparent and require inclusion in the release procedure or become the next area to release.

Within a release position, the therapist sometimes initiates very subtle movements. These movements may be gentle oscillations or involve following a strain pattern in the tissues. Be careful not to move excessively or make any movements without a sense of positive patient response. Some patients find movement irritating to their nervous systems, which may negate the release response.

The proper release position may trigger an intrinsic response or movement on the patient's part, especially if there is trauma in the patient's system. Following these intrinsic movements until their completion will assist the patient in a deeper release of trauma and reorganization of tissues. This has been referred to as *unwinding* by some and should not be inhibited if it occurs.

The release response has been discussed in some depth in Chapter 6, "Patient Participation and Response." To review, the effects of a release can be observed by changes in tissue texture or a decrease in tone and point tenderness. This usually is noted as a melting or softening of the involved tissues. Pulsation or heat also may be observed during or after a release. Occasionally, a tissue response will be triggered that pushes the therapist out of the release position on completion. This usually occurs when there is a history of trauma. Due to the frequently subtle nature of this response, it easily can be missed by a therapist who is not fully aware during the treatment process.

A release can be repeated more than once during a treatment session. If there has been a positive change but you feel that you may be able to effect more change repeat the release, but only two or three times. If a muscle has not released after two or three attempts, either you have not determined the target muscle appropriately, the patient is not responding to this technique, or you need to address a different area before attempting this release.

Remember that the Positional Release descriptions that follow are a general guideline for optimal release of muscles based on anatomical considerations. However, individual variance is the rule. The best results will be obtained by paying attention to palpatory findings of changes in tissue texture and tone and by recreating the patient's unique structural patterns with the releases.

Summary

1. Determine the involved motor units you will treat by using palpation and other evaluation tools.
2. Palpate with gentle pressure in a neutral position to determine point tenderness of trigger point or the area of tissue restriction.

3. Release the pressure but maintain contact with the target tissue as you take the patient into the release position.
4. Take patient slowly into the release position with support and use of the patient's breathing.
5. Palpate the target tissues again, once in the release position, to determine ideal positioning.
6. Reposition, if necessary.
7. Fine tune the release through rotation, longitudinal compression, or distraction.
8. Hold release position for 60–90 seconds or until you palpate a release.
9. Allow for the dynamic release process as needed.
10. Perform isometrics, as needed, from release position.
11. Return the patient to the neutral resting position slowly and passively with support.
12. Reassess target areas with gentle pressure for point tenderness and changes in tone. Repeat other tests, as needed.
13. Repeat the entire process, if needed.

References

1. Juhan D. *Job's Body: A Handbook for Bodywork.* Barrytown, NY: Station Hill Press; 1987:113–114.
2. Gray H, edited by Goss CM. *Gray's Anatomy of the Human Body.* 29th ed. Philadelphia: Lea & Febiger; 1973.
3. Jones LH with Kusunose RS, Goering EK. *Jones Strain-CounterStrain.* Boise, ID: Jones Strain-CounterStrain; 1995.

8

Pelvis and Lower Extremities Muscular Application

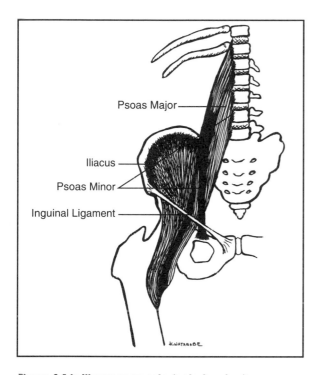

Figure 8-1A: Iliopsoas muscle (anterior view).

The psoas major originates from the anterior bodies, transverse processes, and intervertebral discs of the lumbar vertebrae and inserts into the lesser trochanter of the femur. The iliacus arises from the iliac fossa and crest, base of sacrum, ASIS (anterior superior iliac spine), and AIIS (anterior inferior iliac spine) and is inserted into the lesser trochanter lateral to the psoas tendon.[1] The psoas major passes through the medial arcuate ligament of the diaphragm muscle with the sympathetic chain (see Figure 9-1). The psoas, quadratus lumborum, and the diaphragm share a common fascial arrangement; and therefore all three muscles need to be considered in patients with lumbar and thoracic spine problems, rib dysfunctions, and breathing difficulties.

An arm-length test is used in addition to palpation for the psoas, as a restricted psoas muscle will pull the entire shoulder girdle and trunk complex inferior and result in a short arm side. The patient is supine. The therapist stands on the involved side. Flex the hip and knee to approximately 90° with hip external rotation. Support the leg on therapist's leg or arm. One hand palpates psoas using layer palpation. This release can be done with involved leg only or with both legs bent and supported, if a rotational strain pattern is present throughout pelvis. Add a superior lift on lesser trochanter to facilitate the release as necessary.

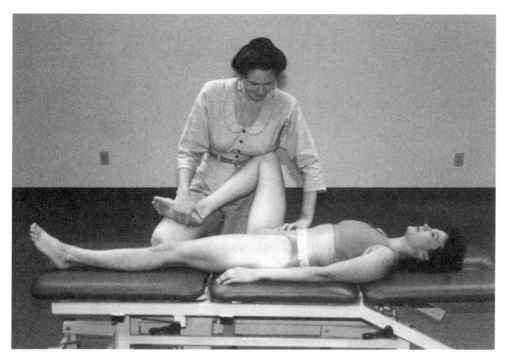

Figure 8-1B: Psoas release.

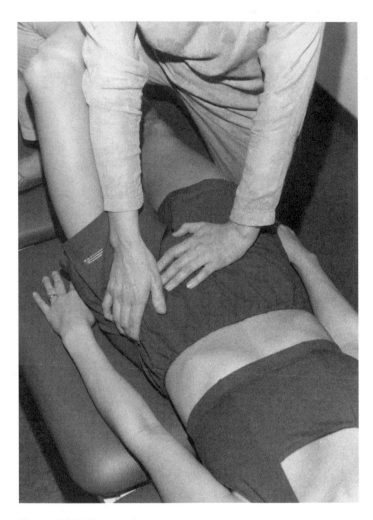

The patient is supine. The therapist stands opposite the involved side. One hand palpates fibers inside the iliac crest. Support involved leg on the therapist's leg with hip and knee flexion and hip external rotation. The other hand brings the iliac crest medial and inferior toward the insertion at the lesser trochanter.

Figure 8-1C: Iliacus release.

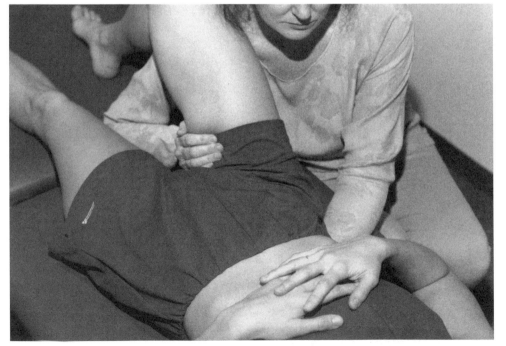

The patient is supine with the involved side hip and knee flexed and the foot resting on the table. The therapist sits on patient's involved side with the knee resting on his or her shoulder. The hip is rotated externally. One hand lifts the lumbar spine transverse processes anterior and inferior while the other hand lifts the lesser trochanter in a superior direction.

Figure 8-1D: Psoas release with the therapist sitting.

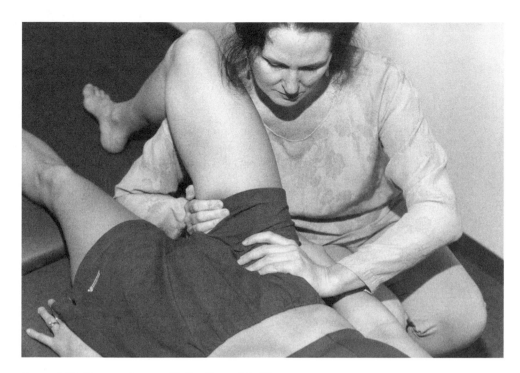

Figure 8-1E: Iliacus release with the therapist sitting.

The patient is supine with the involved side hip and knee flexed and the foot resting on the table. The therapist sits on patient's involved side with the knee resting on his or her shoulder. The hip is externally rotated. One hand lifts the lesser trochanter in a superior direction, while the other hand brings the iliac crest inferior and medial, toward the insertion.

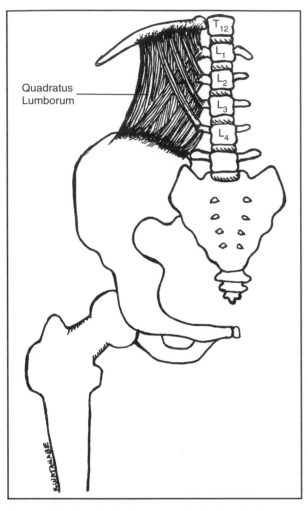

Figure 8-2A: Quadratus lumborum (anterior view).

The quadratus lumborum arises from the iliolumbar ligament and the iliac crest and is inserted into the inferior border of the twelfth rib and to the transverse processes of L_1 through L_4 by four small tendons.[1]

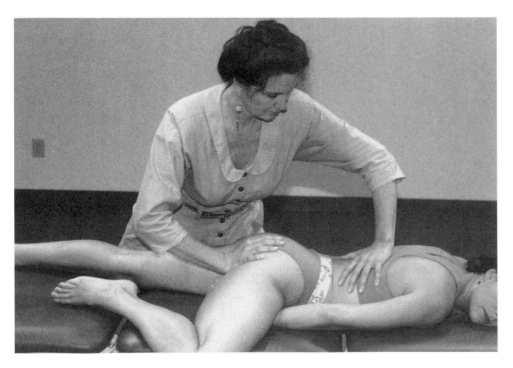

Figure 8-2B: Prone quadratus lumborum release.

The patient is prone. The therapist stands on the involved side. The hip and knee are positioned in flexion, abduction, and side bending toward the involved side with the arm slid under the space between the hip and table. One hand palpates as the other hand takes the lower ribs inferior, the iliac crest superior, or both. You may need to sacrifice your palpating hand to address both components at once. Follow the rotational pattern through the ribs and pelvis to fine tune the release. Patients often report sleeping in a variation of this release position, which chronically shortens the muscle. Use this position for a self-release (see Chapter 5).

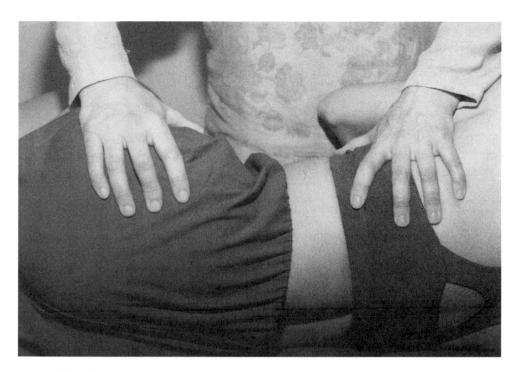

Figure 8-2C: Side-lying quadratus lumborum release.

The patient lies on the uninvolved side. The therapist stands either in front of or behind the patient, supporting the patient's head with a pillow. Bring the lower ribs inferior while taking iliac crest superior. The side bending component happens automatically in side-lying position and the rotational pattern is easier to follow in this position as well.

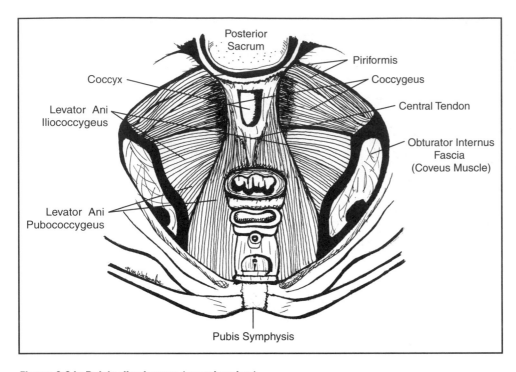

Figure 8-3A: Pelvic diaphragm (superior view).

The pelvic diaphragm is composed of the levator ani and coccygeus muscles. The anterior aspect of the levator ani arises from the superior inner surface of the pubic ramus and the posterior aspect arises from the spine of the ischium and, between these two points, from the fascia of the obturator internus. The two sides of the levator ani inserts into the midline central tendon of the perineum, the sphincter ani, and the last two segments of the coccyx. The levator ani is divided into an anterior aspect (pubococcygeus), which is addressed in the anterior urogenital triangle release, and the posterior aspect (iliococcygeus), which is addressed in the posterior anal triangle release. The coccygeus, which also is part of the posterior triangle, arises from the spine of the ischium and the sacrospinous ligament and inserts into the coccyx and last sacral segment.[1]

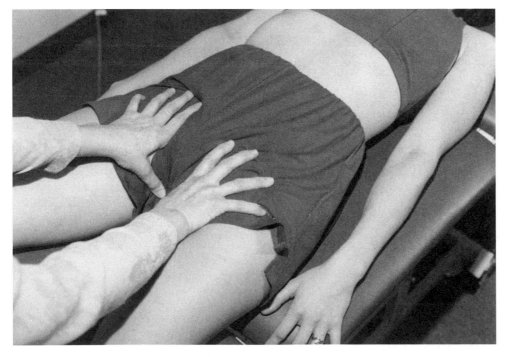

Figure 8-3B: Anterior urogenital triangle release.

The patient is supine, with the legs slightly abducted. The therapist stands at the end of the table. The patient moves closer to the end of the table, so that the therapist is in a comfortable working position with arms extended. The therapist uses a bilateral handhold on the lesser trochanters and if able along the pubic ramus. Take the hips into internal rotation to shorten the anterior fibers of levator ani. Follow any strain present to recreate the patient's unique pattern. Considering doing a hip adductor release first if the lesser trochanter area is too involved to tolerate this pelvic floor release (see Figure 8-7B).

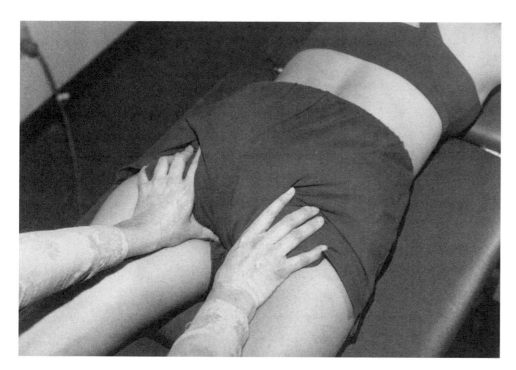

Figure 8-3C: Posterior anal triangle release.

The patient is prone, with the legs slightly abducted. Therapist stands at the end of the table with arms extended. With a bilateral hand-hold, take the hips into external rotation through medial rotation of the ischial tuberosities. Follow any rotational strain patterns present to release.

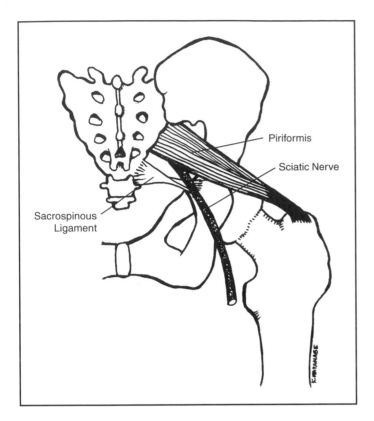

Figure 8-4A: Piriformis (posterior view).

The piriformis arises from the anterior sacrum, sciatic foramen, and the sacrotuberous ligament. It inserts into the greater trochanter of the femur. The sciatic nerve exits the pelvis through the greater sciatic foramen, just below the piriformis muscle. Piriformis spasm can produce pain, numbness, or tingling in the sciatic distribution throughout the posterior leg.[1]

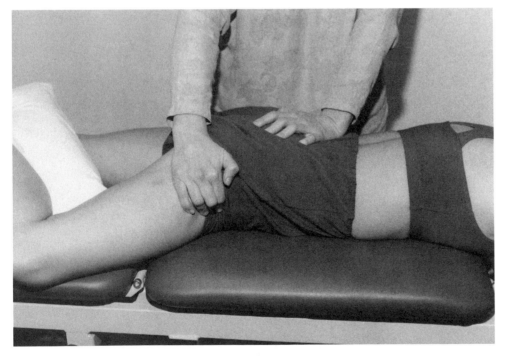

Figure 8-4B: Prone piriformis release.

The patient is prone. The therapist stands opposite the involved side. The hip and knee are flexed with hip external rotation and abduction. One hand blocks the sacral origin and palpates the involved fibers, as the other hand lifts the greater trochanter superior and medial toward the sacrum. The leg can be straight if need be to facilitate the release.

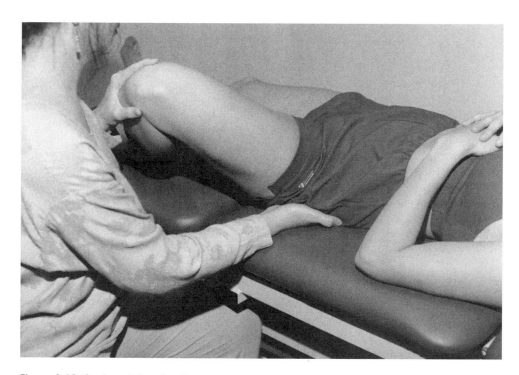

Figure 8-4C: Supine piriformis release.

The patient is supine. The therapist sits on the involved side, with one arm or shoulder supporting the leg. The leg is positioned in hip and knee flexion, using external rotation to fine tune the release. The other hand is under the buttocks, palpating the piriformis. The table serves to passively block the sacrum.

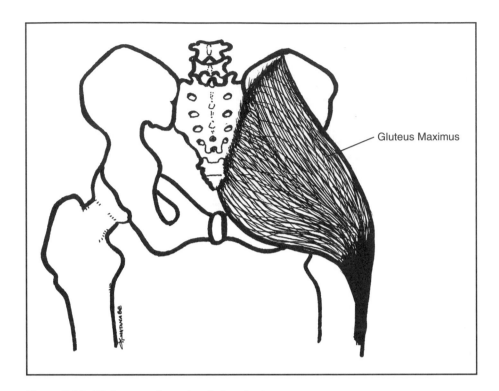

Figure 8-5A: Gluteus maximus (posterior view).

The gluteus maximus has a very broad origin from the ilium, the iliac crest, inferior aspect of the sacrum, and lateral aspect of the coccyx. It also originates from the gluteus medius fascia, the sacrospinalis, and the sacrotuberous ligaments, where fibers intermingle. Insertion is into the posterior femur between the vastus lateralis and adductor magnus tendons and the iliotibial band of the fascia lata.[1]

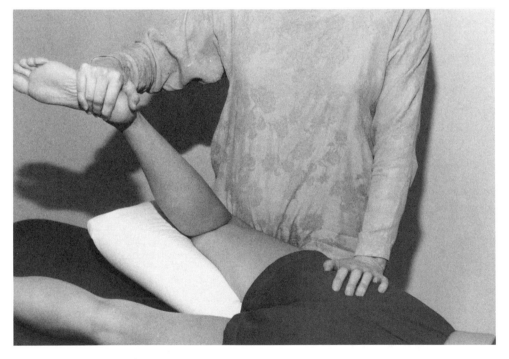

Figure 8-5B: Gluteus maximus release.

Position patient prone. The therapist stands on the involved side. Position involved hip in extension with external rotation and abduction as needed. It is best to position the hip in extension using a pillow, as this allows the therapist to fine tune the release position throughout the entire kinetic chain with an ankle hold. Palpate the involved fibers with your free hand. The gluteus maximus can have many trigger points, which release with slight variations from the basic release position just described. Remember you have nearly 360° freedom of motion at the knee and ankle for position variance.

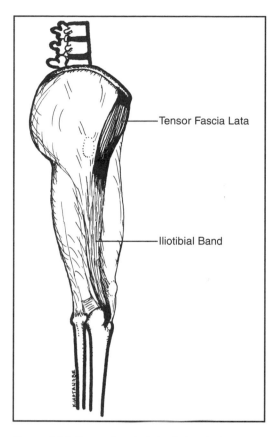

Figure 8-6A: Tensor fascia lata (lateral view).

Tensor Fascia Lata

Iliotibial Band

The tensor fascia lata (TFL) arises from the external aspect of the iliac crest, the ASIS, and the fascia lata. It inserts into the iliotibial band of the fascia lata at the level of the proximal and mid thigh. The iliotibial band continues down the leg to have a broad fascial insertion into the patella.[1]

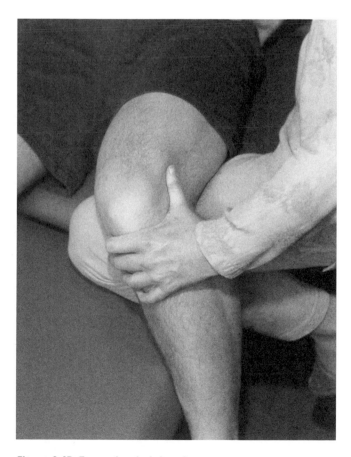

Figure 8-6B: Tensor fascia lata release.

The patient is supine and slides toward the edge of table. The therapist stands on the involved side with the knee bent up on table. The therapist supports the patient's leg on his or her knee with the patient's lower leg off the table. This places the hip in internal rotation. One hand brings iliac crest inferior, as the other hand lifts superior just below mid thigh insertion. To address the entire fascial insertion as shown, take the patella and tibia into a lateral rotation. Use a pillow for positioning, if therapist is unable to tolerate the knee on the table due to patient size, table height, or other considerations. To address the extensive fascial component, deeper work may be required. See the Chapter 5 section, "Integration with Other Techniques."

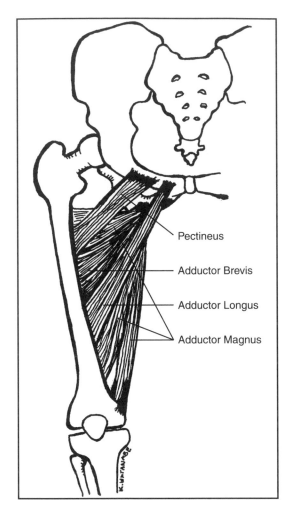

Figure 8-7A: Hip adductors: magnus, longus, and brevis (anterior view).

The hip adductors include the adductor magnus, longus and brevis as well as the pectineus and gracilis. The adductor magnus arises from the inferior pubic ramus, inferior ischial ramus, and the ischial tuberosity and is inserted into the linea aspera along the medial aspect of the entire length of the femur, from the lesser trochanter to the medial condyle. The adductor longus arises from the anterior pubis and inserts into the linea aspera superficial to the magnus in the mid thigh. The adductor brevis arises from the inferior ramus of the pubis and inserts into a line between the lesser trochanter and the linea aspera posterior to the longus.[1]

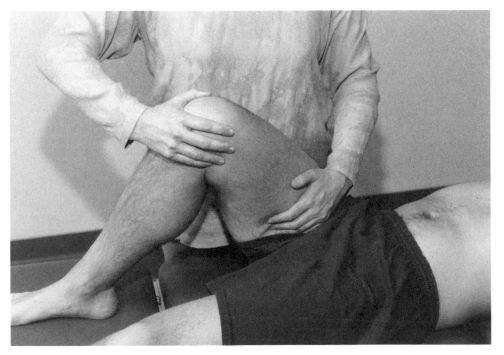

Figure 8-7B: Hip adductor release.

The patient is supine with the involved hip and knee bent and the foot resting on the table. The therapist stands on the involved side. Take the leg into adduction as you fine tune the release through the knee by medially rotating the femur. The foot can be supported on therapist's bent knee or on a pillow, if more hip flexion is needed. The other hand palpates the muscle. Add a superior lift of adductor muscles toward the lesser trochanter and pubis, if necessary. The area around the lesser trochanter can be quite tender to palpation. The adductor release may need to be done prior to other releases that involve manipulation of the lesser trochanter (see Figures 8-1B,D,E and 8-3B). The hip adductor release is excellent for palpating the softening of the tissue tension. As you slowly take the leg into adduction, you can feel the tone decrease through palpation.

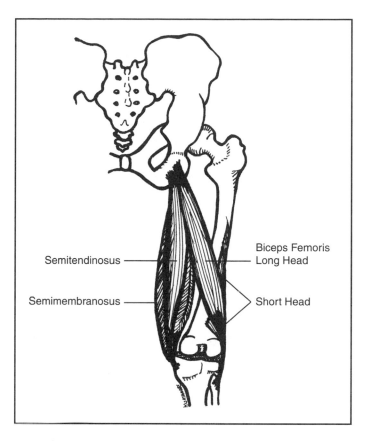

Figure 8-8A: Hamstring muscles (posterior view).

The three hamstring muscles are the lateral biceps femoris and two medial muscles, semitendinosus and semimembranosus. The long head of the biceps femoris arises from the ischial tuberosity and sacrotuberous ligament, while the short head arises from the linea aspera posterior to the adductor magnus. The biceps femoris inserts into the fibular head and the lateral condyle of the tibia. The semitendinosus arises from the ischial tuberosity in common with the biceps femoris and inserts into the medial aspect of the body of the tibia and the deep fascia of the leg. The semimembranosus also arises from the proximal aspect of the ischial tuberosity (separate from the other two hamstrings) and inserts into the lateral condyle of the femur, the fascia of the popliteus muscle, the medial collateral ligament, and fascia of the leg.[1]

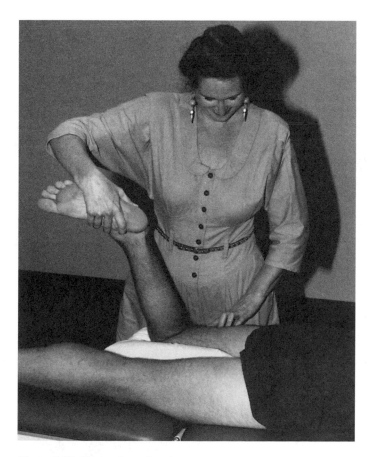

Figure 8-8B: Biceps femoris release.

The patient is prone. The therapist stands on the involved side. Position the hip in extension with a pillow, if tolerated. Keep the hip in neutral regarding extension, if not tolerated. Take the hip into external rotation with knee flexion and external rotation of tibia. Fine tune the release through the entire kinetic chain via the ankle.

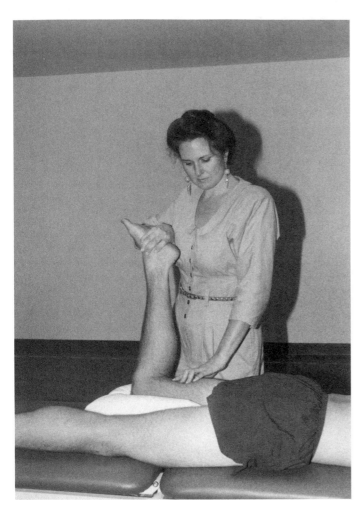

The patient is prone. The therapist stands on the involved side. Position the hip in extension with a pillow, if tolerated. Take the hip into internal rotation with knee flexion and internal rotation of tibia. Fine tune the release through the ankle.

Figure 8-8C: Semitendinosus and semimembranosus release.

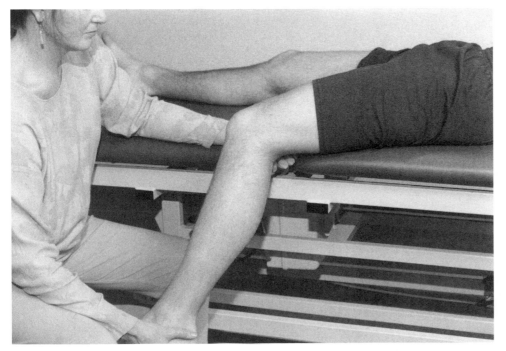

The hamstrings also can be treated effectively with the patient positioned supine. The therapist sits on the involved side on a low stool (or the table is raised). The involved leg is dropped off the table, below the knee. From this position, the therapist can palpate the involved area of the hamstrings with one hand and adjust the position of the hip, knee, and ankle with the other hand. As previously, external rotation of the hip is generally used for the lateral hamstrings and internal rotation for medial hamstrings. The release position often is the same for both medial and lateral hamstrings, in regard to internal or external rotation of the hip, if the patient has a significant strain pattern. Then, only slight variations in ankle movements will be required to fine tune the release.

Figure 8-8D: Hamstring releases with the patient in a supine position.

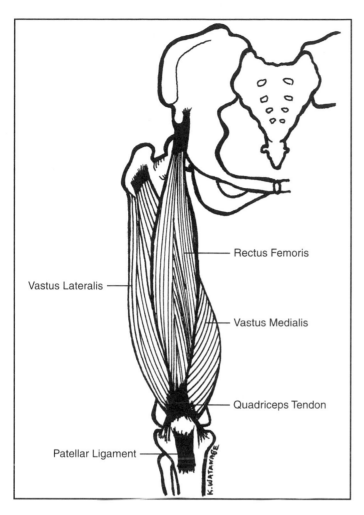

Figure 8-9A: Quadriceps femoris (anterior view).

Labels on figure:
- Rectus Femoris
- Vastus Lateralis
- Vastus Medialis
- Quadriceps Tendon
- Patellar Ligament

Four anterior thigh muscles make up the quadriceps femoris: the rectus femoris, vastus medialis, lateralis, and intermedialis. The rectus femoris arises by two tendons from the AIIS and the brim of the acetabulum and inserts into the base of the patella. The largest part of the quadriceps, the vastus lateralis, arises from a broad aponeurosis attached to the greater trochanter, intertrochanteric line, gluteal tuberosity, linea aspera, gluteus maximus tendon, and lateral intermuscular septum and inserts into the lateral aspect of the patella. The vastus medialis arises from the intertrochanteric line, linea aspera, and medial supracondylar line tendons of the adductor longus and magnus and medial intermuscular septum. It inserts into the medial aspect of the patella. The vastus intermedius arises from the anterior lateral body of the femur and the lateral intermuscular septum, and its fibers form the deep part of the quadriceps tendon.[1]

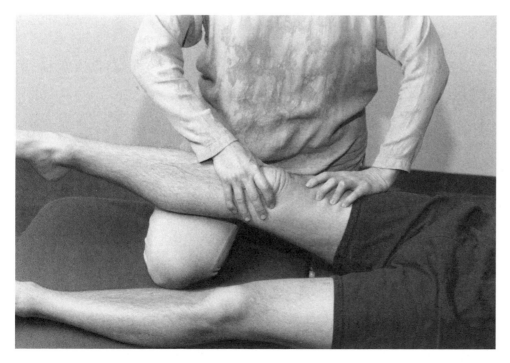

Figure 8-9B: Quadriceps general release.

The patient is supine. The therapist stands on the involved side. The hip is flexed with the knee extended by supporting the straight leg on the therapist's knee (or shoulder, if a more extreme position is required for the release). Support the knee with your hand or a pillow to avoid hyperextension, especially with excessive ligamentous laxity. One hand palpates the muscle while the other lifts the patella superiorly. If the involvement is in the vastus medialis, take the patella more medial; if the involvement is in the vastus lateralis, take the patella more lateral.

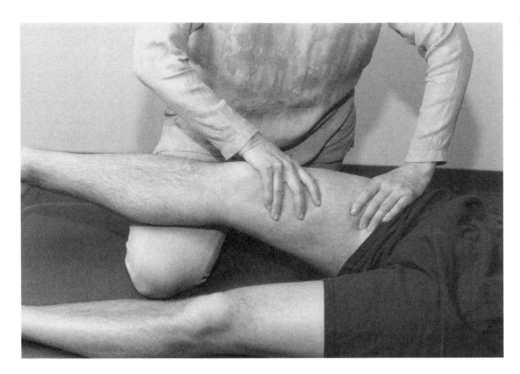

Figure 8-9C: Specific quadriceps releases.

The general release can be modified to treat a more specific dysfunction. A mid muscle release can be done for the most involved fibers (shown). An intermuscular release between the individual quadricep muscles also can be done (not shown). For a rectus femoris origin release, bring the AIIS inferior as you lift patella superior (not shown).

The anterior tibialis arises from the lateral condyle, body of the tibia, interosseous membrane, anterior fascia, intermuscular septum, and extensor digitorum longus. It inserts into the plantar aspect of the first cuneiform and the base of the first metatarsal.[1]

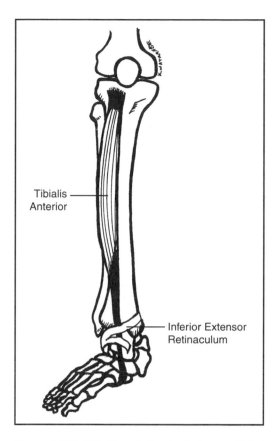

Figure 8-10A: Tibialis anterior (anterior medial view).

The patient is supine. The therapist sits at the end of table. Take the ankle into dorsiflexion and inversion with one hand, while the other hand palpates the muscle. Add rotation through the first metatarsal to fine tune the release.

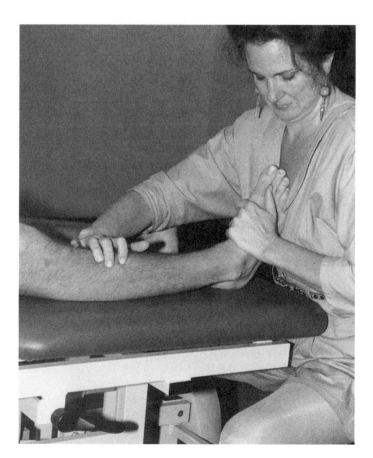

Figure 8-10B: Tibialis anterior release.

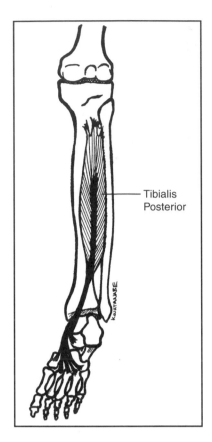

Figure 8-11A: Tibialis posterior (posterior view).

The tibialis posterior arises from the interosseous membrane, intermuscular septum, deep fascia, tibia, and fibula. It inserts into the navicular with slips to the calcaneous, three cuneiforms, cuboid, and second through fourth metatarsal bases.[1] This muscle provides much of the support of the longitudinal arch of the foot.

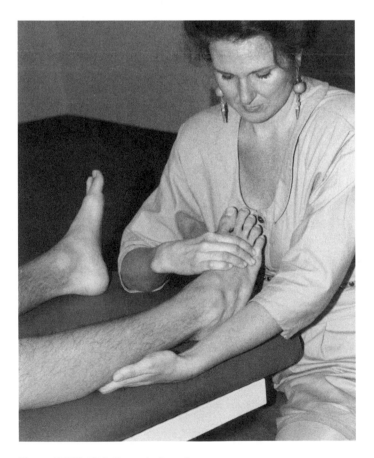

Figure 8-11B: Tibialis posterior release.

The patient is supine. The therapist sits at the end of table. Take the ankle into plantarflexion and inversion. Use layer palpation with other hand. Palpate the tendon posterior to medial malleolus. Add rotation through the metatarsals and navicular to fine tune the release.

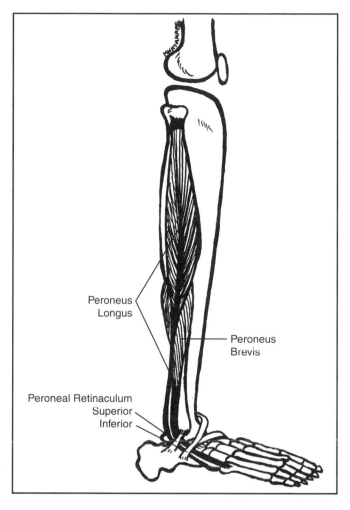

Figure 8-12A: Peroneus longus and brevis (lateral view).

The peroneus longus arises from the fibular head and body, deep fascia, intermuscular septa; and its long tendon runs posterior to the lateral malleolus to insert into the base of the first metatarsal and the medial cuneiform. The peroneus brevis arises from the body of the fibula and intermuscular septa deep to the longus and inserts into the base of the fifth metatarsal bone.[1]

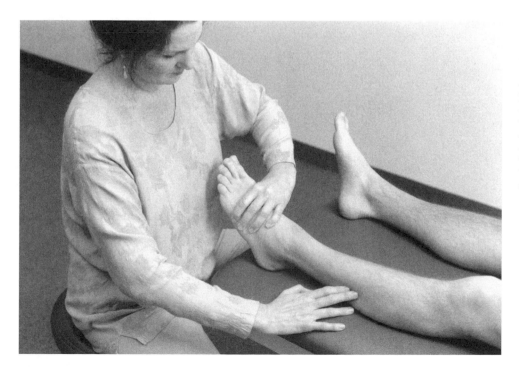

Figure 8-12B: Peroneus longus and brevis release.

The patient is supine. The therapist sits at the end of the table. Take the ankle into plantarflexion and eversion. Palpate muscle with the other hand. Tendons lie posterior to the lateral malleolus. Add rotation through the first metatarsal to fine tune the release with the peroneus longus and use the fifth metatarsal to fine tune the release with the peroneus brevis.

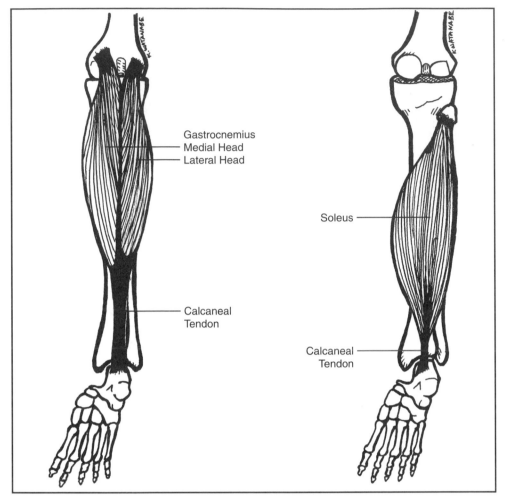

Figure 8-13A: Gastrocnemius (left) and soleus (right) (posterior view).

The gastrocnemius arises by two heads, medial and lateral, from the respective condyles of the femur, the posterior femur, and the knee joint capsule. The tendon joins that of the soleus muscle to form the tendo calcaneus, which inserts into the middle posterior aspect of the calcaneus. The soleus arises deep to the gastrocnemius from the posterior fibula and fibular head and the medial tibia. The tendon joins that of the gastrocnemius muscle to form the tendo calcaneus, which inserts into the medial posterior aspect of the calcaneus.[1]

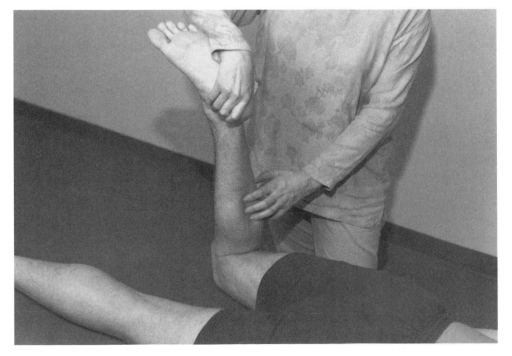

Figure 8-13B: Gastrocnemius and soleus release.

The patient is prone. The therapist stands on the involved side. The knee is flexed to about 90°. One hand plantarflexes the ankle through a hold on the calcaneous, as the other hand palpates the muscle. Use layer palpation for the soleus fibers. Use rotation of calcaneus with inversion and eversion to fine tune the release. Release the calcaneal insertion with inversion or eversion of the calcaneous by approximation between the lower muscle fibers and calcaneous. Release for the soleus muscle is the same except that the knee flexion is not always required for the release.

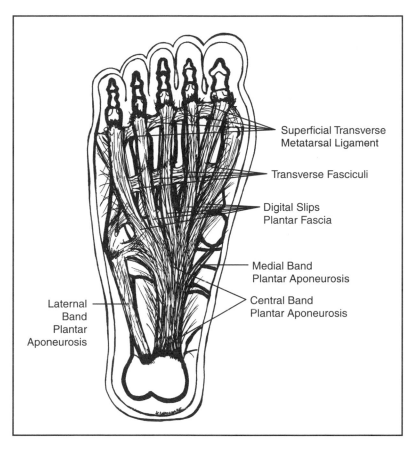

Superficial Transverse
Metatarsal Ligament

Transverse Fasciculi

Digital Slips
Plantar Fascia

Medial Band
Plantar Aponeurosis

Central Band
Plantar Aponeurosis

Laternal
Band
Plantar
Aponeurosis

Figure 8-14A: Plantar fascia (inferior-plantar view).

The plantar fascia is divided into three continuous portions: central, medial, and lateral. The central portion attaches to the calcaneus proximally and divides into five processes to attach to the skin and flexor tendons of each toe. The lateral portion covers the abductor digiti minimi and forms a strong band between the lateral calcaneus and fifth metatarsal. The medial portion covers the abductor hallucis and attaches behind the flexor retinaculum.[1]

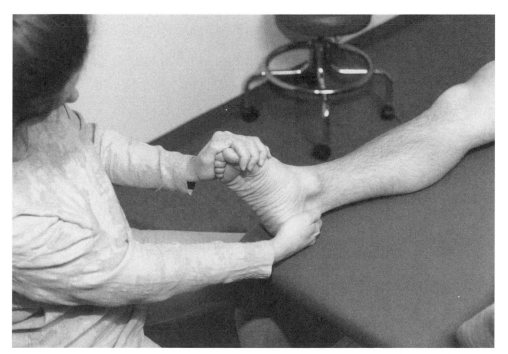

Figure 8-14B: Plantar fascia release.

The patient is supine or prone. The therapist sits at the end of the table. Take the toes and metatarsals into plantarflexion while pulling the calcaneus inferior toward the toes. Fine tune the release with a rotational component. Deeper soft tissue work may be added while in the release position, as necessary. This release is included to demonstrate the application to primarily fascial tissues with secondary muscular relationships.

Reference

1. Gray H; Goss CM, ed. *Gray's Anatomy of the Human Body.* 29th ed. Philadelphia: Lea and Febiger; 1973.

9

Trunk and Upper Extremity Muscular Application

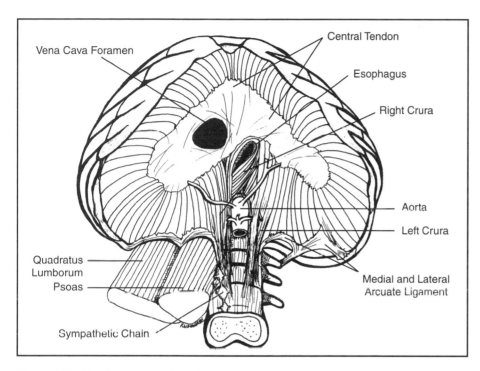

Figure 9-1A: Diaphragm muscle (inferior view).

The diaphragm has three origins. The sternal portion arises by two slips from the xiphoid process. The costal portion arises from the inner side of the last six ribs, their cartilage, and the transverse abdominus. The lumbar portion arises from the anterior aspect of the lumbar vertebrae by two crura. The psoas major muscle and the sympathetic chain pass through the medial arcuate ligament, while the quadratus lumborum passes through the lateral arcuate ligament. The diaphragm insertion is into the central tendon, which is a strong aponeurosis located closer to the anterior aspect of thorax. The diaphragm has three large openings for the aorta, esophagus, and the vena cava.[1]

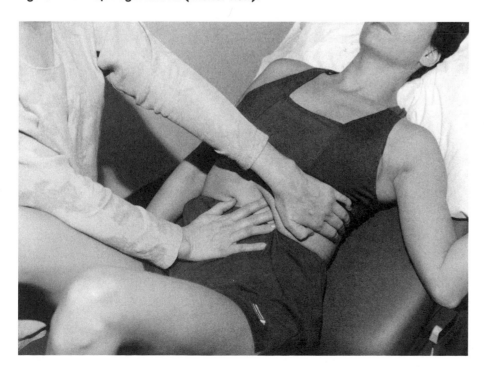

Figure 9-1B: Costal diaphragm release.

The patient is supine with knees bent and feet resting on a table, stool, or pillows for support. The therapist stands opposite the involved side. Palpate under the rib cage on the involved side. Bring the lower ribs inferior and medial toward the palpating hand. If a strain pattern is noted, bring the shoulder inferior and medial, to include entire shoulder girdle in the release. The awareness and use of breathing is important with all releases but especially so with the diaphragm. Have the patient inhale then exhale as you take him or her into the release position. With the diaphragm, you need to maintain some tension on the system during the release, but be careful not to impede the patient's breathing.

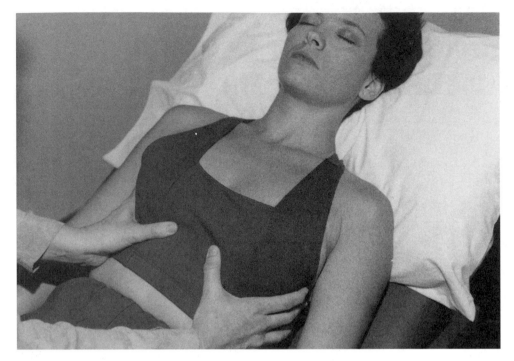

The patient position is the same as in the preceding, the therapist can stand on either side. Hands are placed on the sides of ribs below the breasts with broad surface contact. Take the ribs medial and slightly posterior, toward lumbar spine insertion. This is an excellent release to follow rotational strain patterns through the thorax.

Figure 9-1C: Lateral diaphragm release.

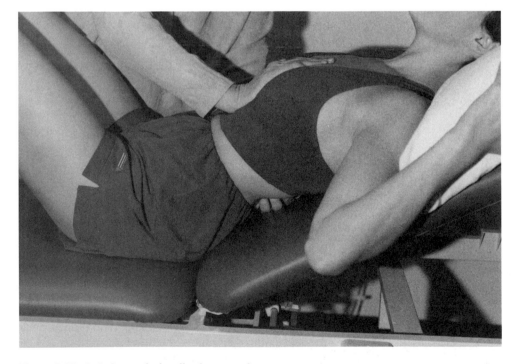

The patient is again supine with knees bent. The therapist stands or sits at either side. One hand tractions the sternum and lower ribs, inferior and posterior, while other hand lifts the transverse processes of upper lumbar vertebrae in an anterior superior direction.

Figure 9-1D: Anterior-posterior diaphragm release.

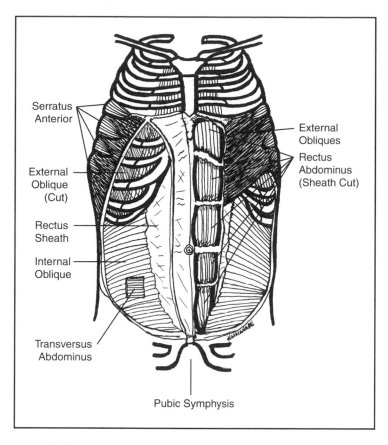

Figure 9-2A: Rectus abdominus (anterior view).

The rectus abdominis arises from a lateral tendon emanating from the pubic bone and a medial tendon from ligaments around the pubis on the same and opposite sides. Insertion is into the cartilages of the fifth, sixth, and seventh ribs. The rectus abdominis muscle is enclosed in a sheath made up of fibers from the external obliques, internal obliques, and transverse abdominis. The linea alba is the mid-line between the two rectus abdominis muscles. It is formed where the fibers of the obliques and transverse abdominis fuse with fibers from the same muscles on the other side.[1]

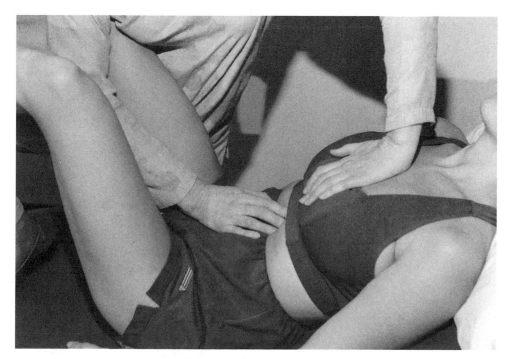

Figure 9-2B: Rectus abdominus release.

The patient is supine. The therapist stands on the involved side. Elevate the trunk by raising the head of the table or positioning with pillows. Flex the patient's knees and hips by positioning on a stool or the therapist's leg (shown). If necessary, you can hyperflex the legs further with one arm while the other hand takes ribs five, six, seven, and the sternum inferior toward the pubic bone. If you have a free hand use it to palpate or take the lower fibers of the muscle toward the rib insertions. The rectus abdominis frequently is involved following abdominal surgery.

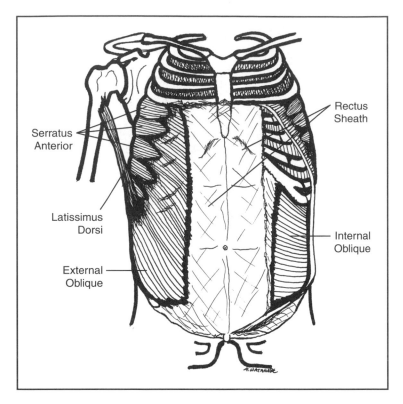

Serratus
Anterior

Latissimus
Dorsi

External
Oblique

Rectus
Sheath

Internal
Oblique

Figure 9-3A: External and internal oblique muscles (anterior view).

The external oblique is more superior and superficial than the internal oblique. The external oblique arises from the lower eight ribs and interdigitates with fibers from the serratus anterior and the latissimus dorsi. The insertion for the externus is into the anterior aspect of the iliac crest and into a broad abdominal aponeurosis that ends in the linea alba. The internal oblique, which is deep to the externus, is a smaller, thinner muscle. It arises from the inguinal ligament, iliac crest, iliac, and thoracolumbar fascia. It inserts into the ninth through twelfth ribs and intercostal muscles and also contributes to the rectus sheath, which terminates in the linea alba.[1]

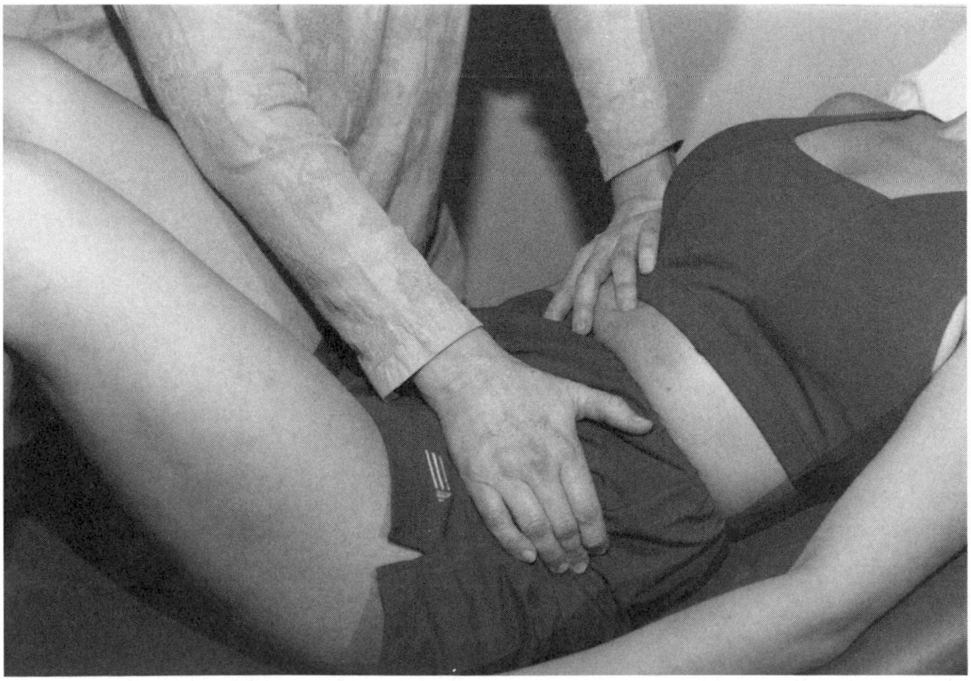

Figure 9-3B: External and internal obliques release.

The patient is supine. The knees are bent and the trunk is elevated, as with the rectus abdominis release. The therapist stands on either side of the patient. This release addresses the external oblique on one side, with the internal oblique on the other side. One hand takes the lower ribs inferior and medial (external oblique), while the other hand takes the iliac crest of the other side superior and medial (internal oblique). This release will address the diagonal strain pattern throughout the trunk. Often there will be a distinct asymmetry between the two sides. It is best to perform a motion test for the preferred pattern and ease of motion with both diagonals to determine the muscle restrictions that need to be addressed.

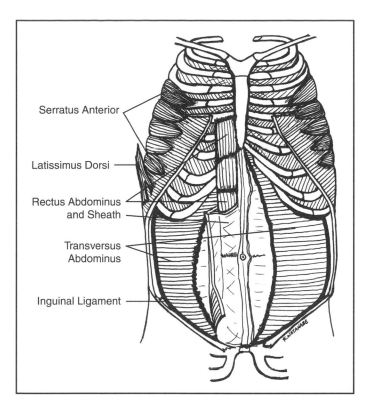

Figure 9-4A: Transversus abdominus muscle (anterior view).

Serratus Anterior

Latissimus Dorsi

Rectus Abdominus and Sheath

Transversus Abdominus

Inguinal Ligament

The transverse abdominus is deep to the internal oblique. Like the internal oblique, this muscle arises from the inquinal ligament, iliac crest and the thoracolumbar fascia. It also arises from the lower six ribs and their cartilage. The fibers cross horizontally to combine with the internal oblique aponeurosis and contribute to the rectus sheath, which terminates in the linea alba.[1]

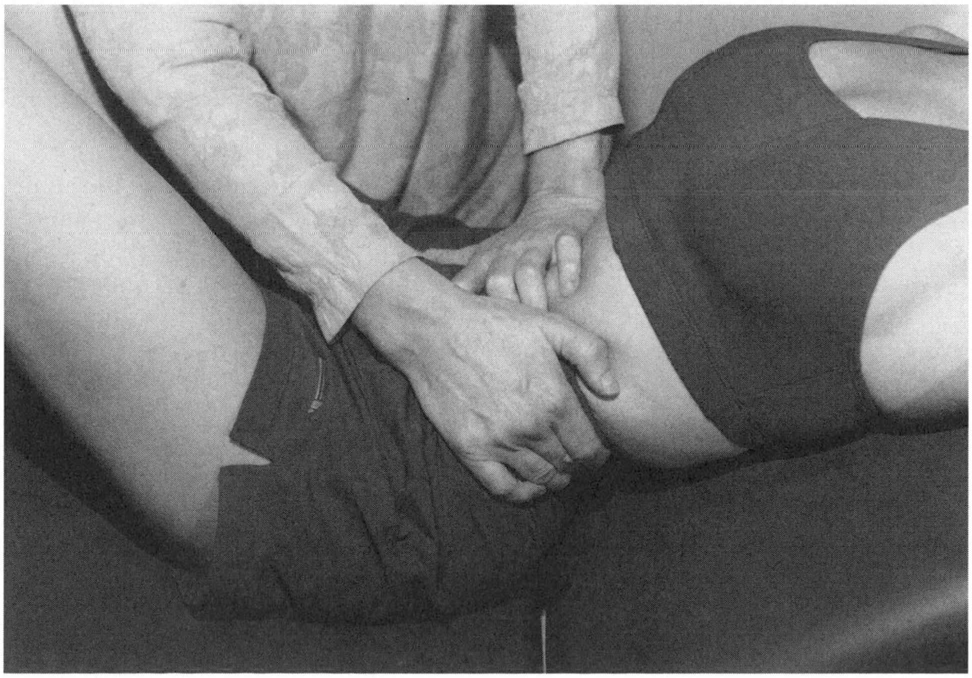

Figure 9-4B: Tranversus abdominus release.

The patient is supine. The therapist stands opposite the involved side. The knees are bent and the trunk is elevated, as with other abdominal muscle releases. Take the rectus abdominis laterally with one hand as you bring the thoracolumbar fascia in a medial and anterior direction with the other hand (shown). The hand that moves the rectus laterally also can palpate the involved fibers. The lower ribs or iliac crest also can be used for the release by taking them medial and anterior toward the rectus, which is moved laterally (not shown). Examination of the abdominal muscles is important, if there has been surgical or other soft tissue trauma to the abdomen. Involvement of the abdominal muscles often will contribute to low back pain.

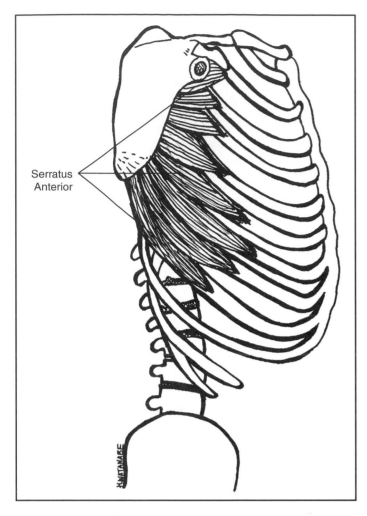

Figure 9-5A: Serratus anterior muscle (lateral view).

The serratus anterior arises from the first eight or nine ribs and their intercostal muscles. The insertion is into the ventral aspect of the scapulae, on the vertebral border from the superior to inferior angle. The origin of the lower four slips interdigitate with the origin of the external oblique muscle.[1]

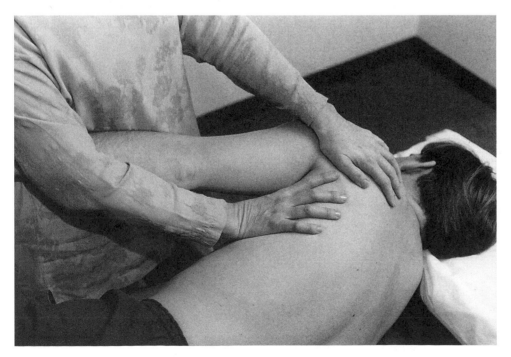

Figure 9-5B: Serratus anterior release.

Position the patient on the uninvolved side. The therapist stands in front of patient. The patient's arm should be elevated and supported either with pillows or on therapist's hip (shown). Take scapula into protraction as you take ribs one through nine posterior and superior toward scapula, with the other hand.

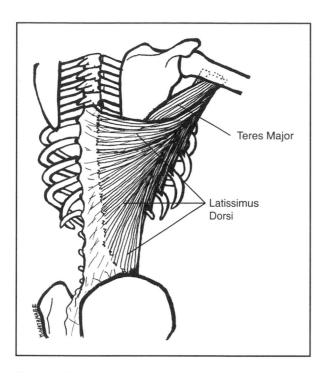

Figure 9-6A: Latissimus dorsi and teres major muscles (posterior-lateral view).

The latissimus dorsi has a very extensive origin, from the lumbar aponeurosis (a layer of the thoracolumar fascia) that attaches to the spinous processes of the sacral and lumbar vertebrae, the lower six thoracic vertebrae, and the supraspinal ligament. It also arises from the posterior aspect of the iliac crest and the lower three or four ribs. A few fasciculi attach the muscle to the scapulae, and as the muscle fibers converge toward the shoulder, they twist upon themselves. The insertion is into the intertubercular groove of the humerus between the teres major tendon (posterior) and the pectoralis major tendon (anterior) with two bursa separating the three tendons.[1]

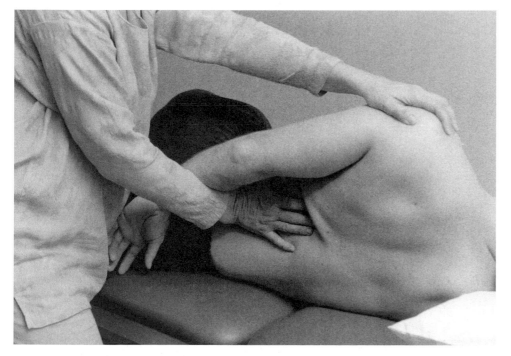

Figure 9-6B: Latissimus dorsi release.

Position the patient on the uninvolved side, with the involved hand resting behind the patient's back (if able to tolerate this). The therapist stands behind the patient. Take the shoulder into increased extension and adduction, if needed, and concentrate on the internal rotation component with a proximal hold on the humerus. Traction the shoulder inferior and medial as the other hand palpates and takes sacrum, lumbar, or thoracic spine superior and lateral toward the shoulder, adjusting the amount of spinal extension.

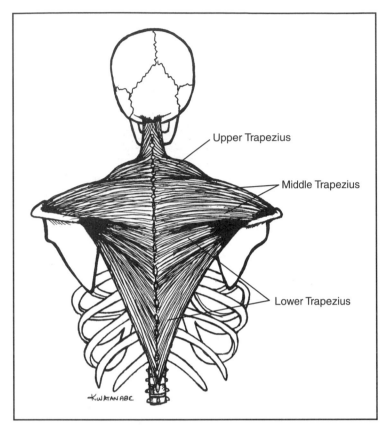

Figure 9-7A: Trapezius muscle (posterior view).

The origin of the trapezius muscle is from the external occipital protuberance, the ligamentum nuchae, the spinous processes of C_7 through T_{12}, and the supraspinal ligament. The upper trapezius fibers insert into the posterior lateral aspect of the clavicle. The middle trapezius fibers insert into the acromium and the superior aspect of the spine of the scapulae. The lower trapezius fibers converge toward the scapulae and insert into the medial end of the spine of the scapulae in a triangular aponeurosis.[1]

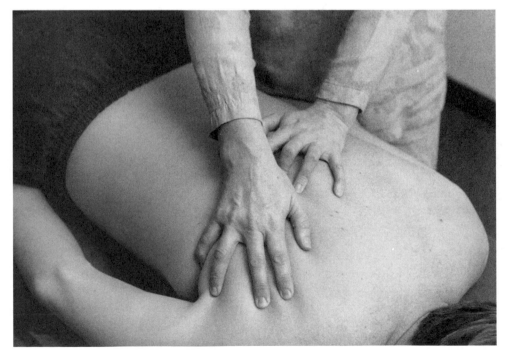

Figure 9-7B: Middle and lower trapezius release.

The patient is prone. The therapist stands opposite the involved side. Take the scapula medial toward spinal origin with one hand. The other hand blocks at the spine and palpates the involved fibers. Vary the angle of pull and adjust your standing position to line up your arms with the direction of the fibers. For the lower trapezius, first rotate the inferior angle of scapula in a lateral direction then take it inferior and medial toward the spine to release (shown). For the middle trapezius fibers, a straight medial pull would be required with a lift from the spine of the scapula for a more specific release.

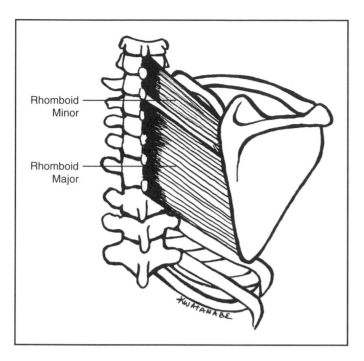

Figure 9-8A: Rhomboid major and minor muscles (posterior view).

The rhomboid major arises from the spinous processes of T_2 through T_5 and the supraspinal ligament. The insertion is into the vertebral border of the scapulae by a tendinous arch. The rhomboid minor arises from the spinous processes of C_7 through T_1 and the inferior portion of the ligamentum nuchae. It is inserted into the root of the spine of the scapulae.[1]

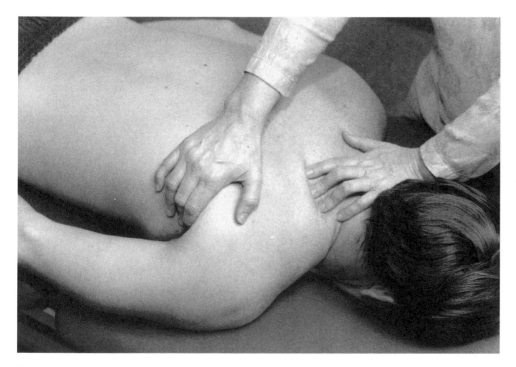

Figure 9-8B: Rhomboid major and minor release.

The patient is prone. The therapist stands opposite the involved side, toward the head of the table. Take the scapula medial and superior into elevation. The other hand can block spinal insertions at C_7 through T_5 and palpate. With this and all prone releases, unless indicated otherwise, either use a face cradle or have the head turned toward the side you are lifting.

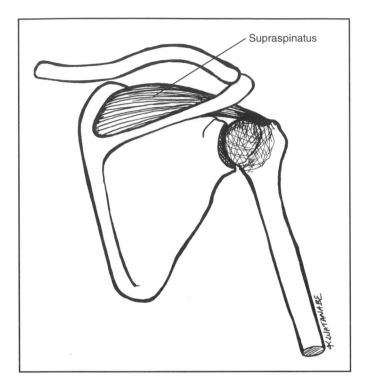

Figure 9-9A: Supraspinatus muscle (posterior view).

The supraspinatus arises from the medial two thirds of supraspinatus fossa and its fascia. The muscle fibers insert into the greater tubercle of the humerus superior to the infraspinatus tendon. Fibers from this tendon go into the shoulder joint capsule.[1]

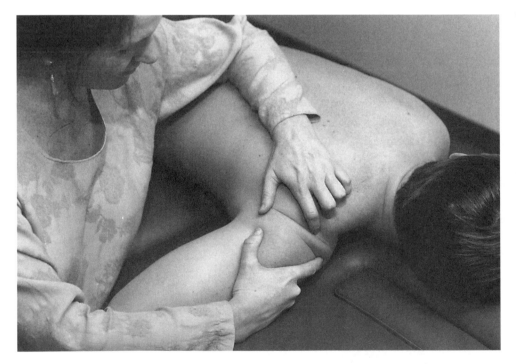

Figure 9-9B: Supraspinatus release.

The patient is prone. The therapist sits on the involved side. The involved arm below the elbow is off the table with the upper arm supported by the table in a neutral position (regarding rotation). Approximate the humerus toward the scapula. The other hand palpates and approximates the scapula toward the humerus. This also can be done with patient in a supine position, but the arm will require more support from the therapist or a pillow in that position.

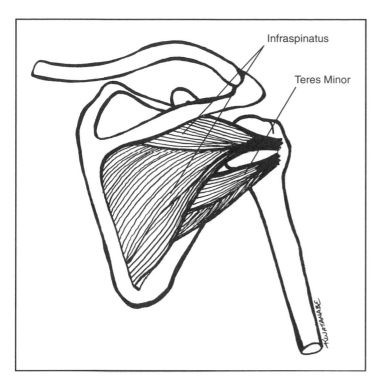

Figure 9-10A: Infraspinatus and teres minor muscles (posterior view).

The infraspinatus arises from the infraspinatous fossa and fascia of the scapulae and inserts into the greater tubercle of the humerus between the supraspinatous and the teres minor tendons, to which it is fused. The teres minor arises from the posterior lateral border of the scapulae between the infraspinatus and the teres major muscles, which contribute to its origin through aponeurotic laminae. It inserts into the inferior aspect of the greater tubercle of the humerus, and its fibers contribute to the posterior aspect of the shoulder joint capsule.[1]

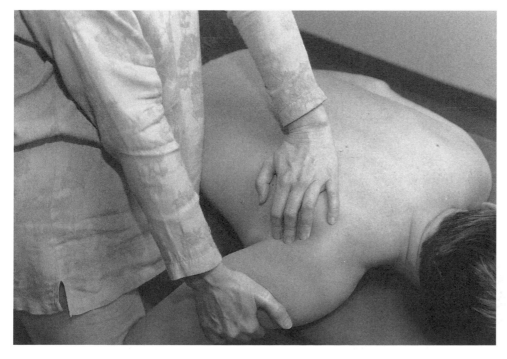

Figure 9-10B: Infraspinatus and teres minor release.

The patient is prone with the involved arm off table, close to the edge of the table. The therapist stands on the involved side. Take the shoulder into slight extension with external rotation (with the elbow flexion) with one hand, while the other hand takes the scapula into protraction and palpates the involved fibers. The first hand adjusts the amount of shoulder external rotation to fine tune the release. You may need to drop the shoulder off the table as well if a forward shoulder is present. This release also can be done in the side-lying and supine positions.

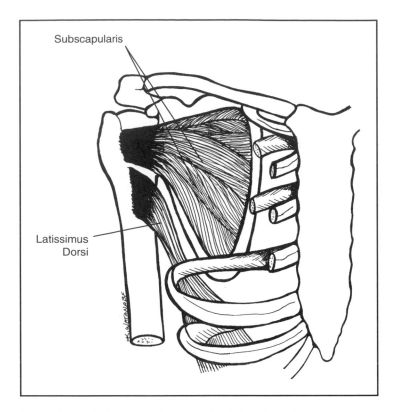

Figure 9-11A: Subscapularis muscle (anterior view, ribs cut).

The subscapularis arises from the subcapularis fossa and fascia of the scapulae and from the aponeurotic laminae from the teres major and the long head of the triceps. It inserts into the lesser tubercle of the humerus and the anterior shoulder joint capsule. (See Figure 9-6 for a posterior view of the teres major.) The teres major arises from the posterior surface of the inferior angle of the scapulae and inserts into the lesser tubercle of the humerus, posterior to the latissimus dorsi, with their fibers united for a short distance.[1]

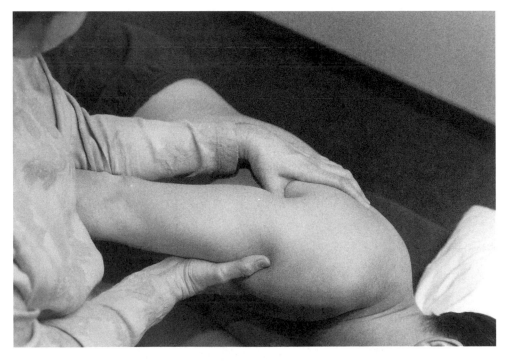

Figure 9-11B: Subscapularis and teres major release.

The patient lies on the uninvolved side. The therapist stands in front of the patient. Extend the arm and support it on therapist's hip or on pillows. One hand takes the scapula into protraction and palpates the muscle fibers under scapula with the thumb. The other hand takes the shoulder into internal rotation to fine tune the release.

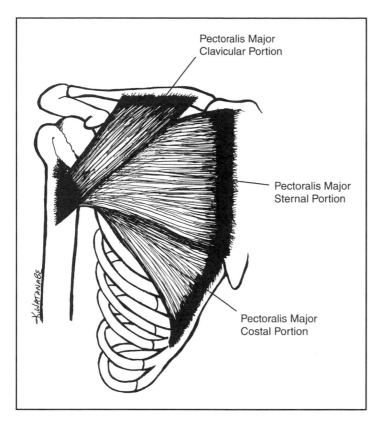

Figure 9-12A: Pectoralis major muscle (anterior view).

The pectoralis major arises from the medial half of the clavicle, the anterior surface of the sternum, the cartilage of the first six or seven ribs, and the external oblique aponeurosis. The fibers converge toward the insertion on the greater tubercle of the humerus by two lamina. The anterior lamina contains fibers from the clavicular portion of the muscle and the superior sternal fibers. The posterior lamina is the attachment for most of the sternal and the costal portion of the muscle.[1]

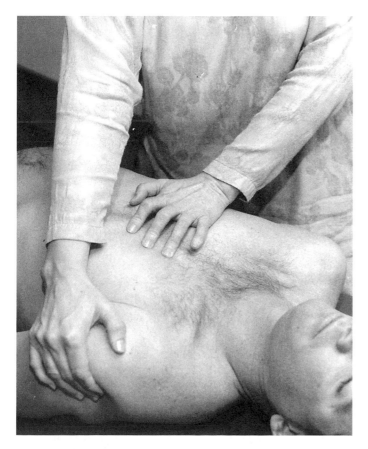

Figure 9-12B: Sternal and costal releases.

The patient is supine. The therapist stands opposite the involved side. The arm rests at the patient's side in an internal rotation (palm down). Take the shoulder medial and inferior for costal and sternal releases. The other hand blocks at sternum and palpates. The angle of pull will vary according to the muscle fibers you are targeting to release.

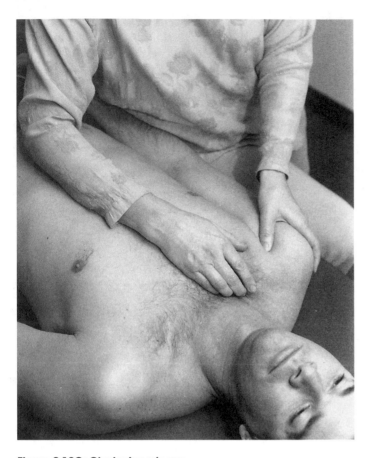

Figure 9-12C: Clavicular release.

The patient is supine. The therapist stands on the involved side. One hand palpates the clavicular portion of the muscle as you take the clavicle inferior and lateral, if patient is able to tolerate the pressure on the clavicle. Use your hand in a broad surface contact. The other hand rotates the shoulder internally and takes it in a superior and medial direction toward the clavicle.

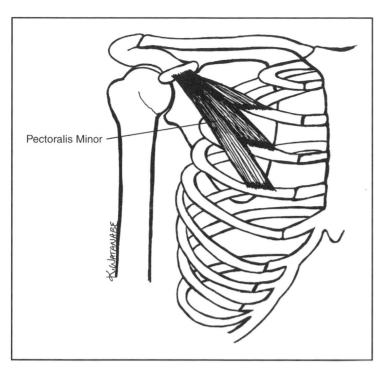

Figure 9-13A: Pectoralis minor muscle (anterior view).

The pectoralis minor arises from the third, fourth, and fifth ribs and their intercostal muscles and inserts into the medial and superior aspect of the coracoid process of the scapulae.[1]

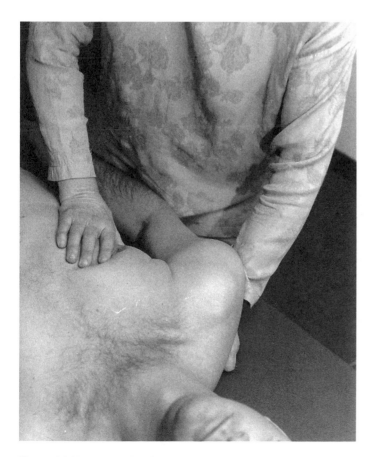

Figure 9-13B: Pectoralis minor release.

The patient is supine. The therapist stands or sits on the involved side. Palpate the pectoralis minor fibers under the pectoralis major. Bring the scapula (coracoid process) anterior and inferior toward the upper ribs. Elevate ribs three, four, and five toward the coracoid process. The scapula can be positioned as just described using a towel roll (not shown). This will free your other hand for palpation, which is difficult under the pectoralis major. Examination of this muscle is very important for upper extremity dysfunction, especially with thoracic outlet syndrome and reflex sympathetic dystrophy.

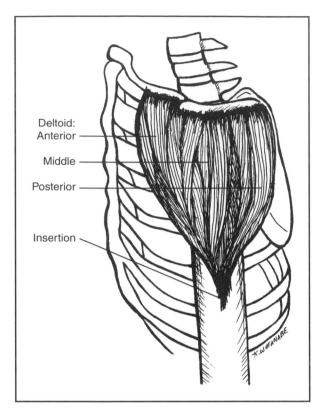

Figure 9-14A: Deltoid muscle (lateral view).

The deltoid arises from the anterior aspect of the lateral third of the clavicle, the acromion process, and the posterior border of the spine of the scapulae. The insertion is by a thick tendon on the lateral body of the humerus (deltoid prominence) and into the fascia of the arm.[1]

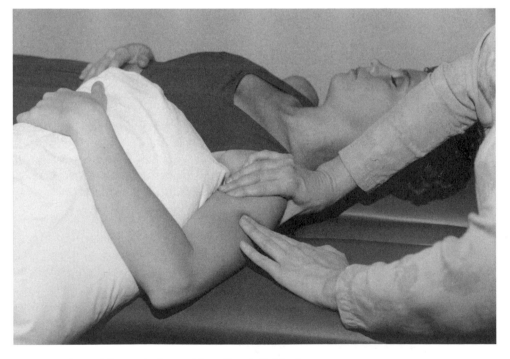

Figure 9-14B: Middle, posterior, and insertion deltoid releases.

The patient is supine. The therapist sits on the involved side. The arm is positioned in approximately 90° of abduction with a neutral rotation. The therapist can support the arm in this position with one hand or use pillows. For the middle deltoid, approximate fibers toward the scapular origin and palpate with either hand as able (not shown). Release the posterior deltoid as the middle deltoid, except with shoulder in external rotation and extension by dropping the arm off the table if needed (not shown). Release the deltoid insertion in a similar position, by taking the fibers of the muscle inferior toward the humerus (shown).

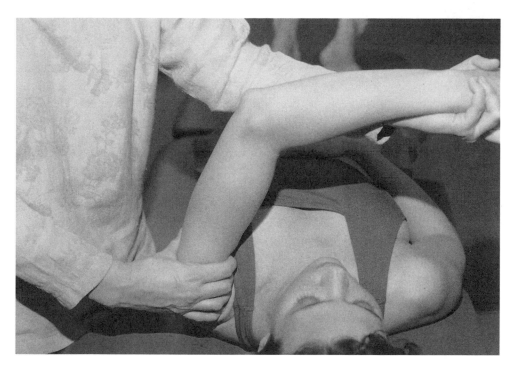

Figure 9-14C: Anterior deltoid release.

The patient is supine with 90° of abduction. For the anterior deltoid, the therapist should stand on the involved side and take the arm into a horizontal adduction with the shoulder in internal rotation.

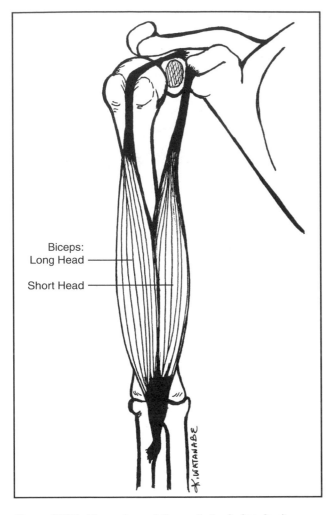

Figure 9-15A: Biceps branchii muscle (anterior view).

Biceps:
Long Head
Short Head

The short head of the biceps arises from the apex of the coracoid process of the scapulae, along with the coracobrachialis. The long head arises from the supraglenoid tuberosity of the scapulae, above the glenoid fossa. The long head of the biceps tendon is enclosed in a synovial sheath and is part of the joint capsule, until it exits into the bicipital groove. The biceps inserts into the radial tuberosity.[1]

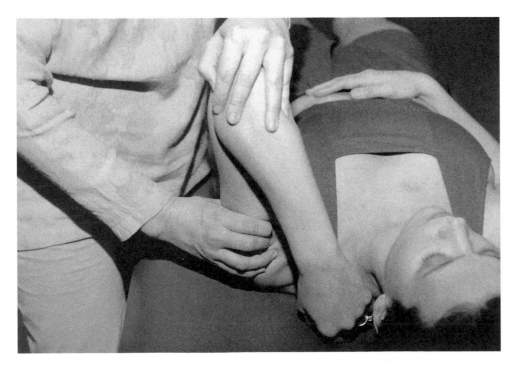

Figure 9-15B: Biceps branchii release.

The patient is supine. The therapist stands on the involved side. The arm should be in a position of shoulder and elbow flexion with supination at the forearm. The shoulder is abducted and externally rotated (generally in a hand to ear position). The therapist positions the patient and fine tunes the release with one hand as the other hand palpates the involved fibers.

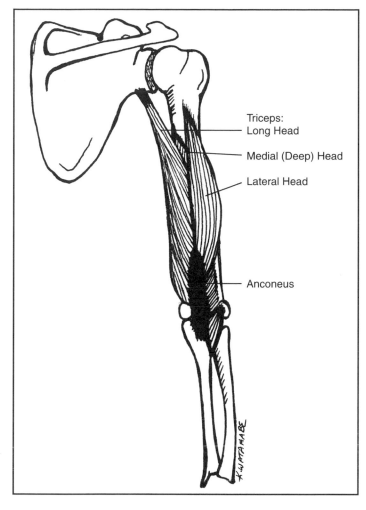

Figure 9-16A: Triceps branchii and anconeus muscles (posterior view).

The long head of the triceps originates from the infraglenoid tuberosity of the scapulae, just below the glenoid fossa. The medial (deep) head has a broad origin from the posterior and medial aspect of the humerus just below the groove for the radial nerve and the intermuscular septum. The lateral head also arises from the humerus proximal and superficial to the medial head. The triceps inserts into the olecranon, anconeus, and deep fascia of the forearm. The anconeus arises from the lateral epicondyle of the humerus just below the medial head of the triceps and inserts into the olecranon and shaft of the ulna.[1]

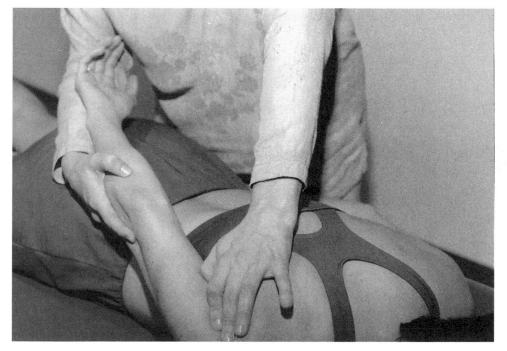

Figure 9-16B: Triceps branchii and anconeus release.

Position the patient prone. The therapist stands opposite involved side. Take the arm into extension at shoulder and elbow with some shoulder adduction. Do not lock the elbow in extension. This position will address the long head of triceps as well as the medial and lateral heads. The triceps release can be done with the patient supine and the arm off the table in shoulder extension; however, the adduction component (for the long head) is difficult to create in this position. The anconeus can be similarly released with the patient supine or prone, with more focus on fine-tuning the release distal to the elbow joint (not shown).

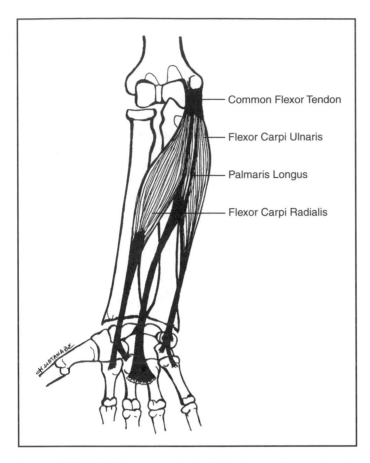

Figure 9-17A: Wrist flexor muscle (anterior view, palmar surface).

The common flexor tendon arises from the medial epicondyle of the humerus. This gives rise to the three superficial flexor muscles of the forearm shown: flexor carpi radialis, palmaris longus, and flexor carpi ulnaris. The deeper wrist flexors include flexor digitorum superficialis and profundus and flexor pollicus longus. The pronator teres should be considered in the release; however, it does not flex the wrist.[1]

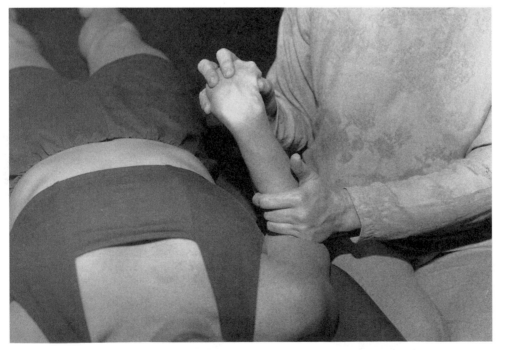

Figure 9-17B: Wrist flexor release.

The patient is supine. The therapist sits on the involved side. A general release of the superficial wrist flexor group is with 90° or more of elbow flexion and wrist and finger flexion. Pronation of the elbow is included in the release because of the pronator teres association at the origin. The deeper wrist and finger flexors (flexor digitorum profundus and flexor pollicis longus—not shown) can be released with a more neutral position of the elbow and a focus on wrist and finger flexion. Adjust pronation, supination, radial and ulnar deviation, and the degree of flexion to fine tune the release.

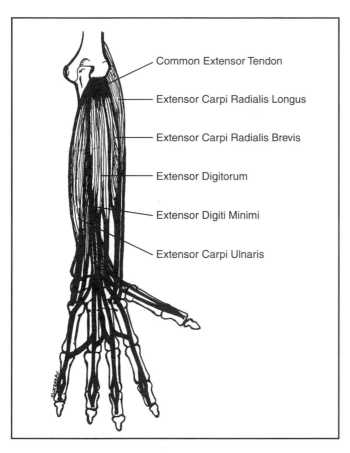

Figure 9-18A: Wrist extensor muscle (posterior view).

The common extensor tendon arises from the lateral epicondyle of the humerus. This gives rise to the four wrist extensors shown: extensor carpi radialis brevis, extensor digitorum, extensor digiti minimi, and extensor carpi ulnaris. The extensor carpi radialis longus muscle (also shown) arises from the humerus just above the common extensor tendon. The supinator muscle (not shown) also arises from a broad origin on the lateral epicondyle of the humerus and should be considered in the release but does not extend the wrist.[1]

The labels in the figure, from top to bottom:

- Common Extensor Tendon
- Extensor Carpi Radialis Longus
- Extensor Carpi Radialis Brevis
- Extensor Digitorum
- Extensor Digiti Minimi
- Extensor Carpi Ulnaris

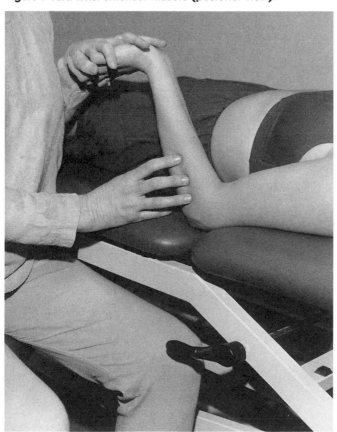

Figure 9-18B: Wrist extensor release.

The patient is supine. The therapist sits on the involved side. A general release of the wrist extensor group is with elbow supination and wrist and finger extension. Regarding flexion and extension, the elbow is in a neutral position. Adjust supination, pronation, radial, and ulnar deviation and the amount of extension in wrist and fingers to fine tune the release.

Reference

1. Gray H; Goss CM, ed. *Gray's Anatomy of the Human Body.* 29th ed. Philadelphia: Lea and Febiger; 1973.

10

Head and Neck Muscular Application

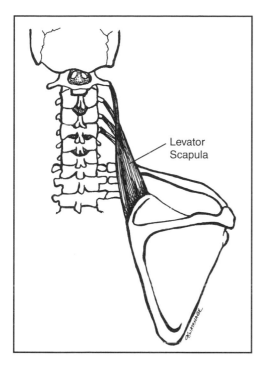

Figure 10-1A: Levator scapula muscle (posterior view).

The levator scapula muscle arises from the transverse processes of C_1 through C_4. The muscle fibers twist slightly as they approach the insertion into the superior angle of the scapula along the vertebral border.[1]

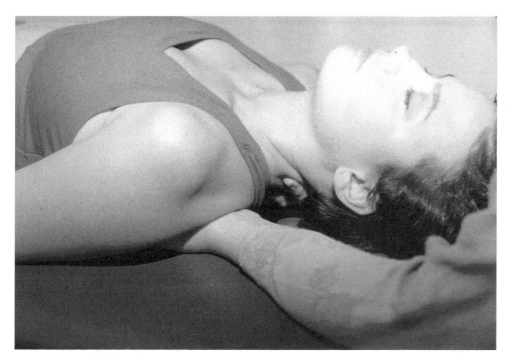

Figure 10-1B: Levator scapula release.

The patient is supine. The therapist sits at the head of the table. One hand palpates and controls a slight neck rotation to the same side. The other hand slides under the scapula with fingertips below the inferior angle. Traction the scapula into elevation toward insertion at the C_1 through C_4 transverse processes. The release can be done with the patient in a prone position but the neck position is difficult to fine tune.

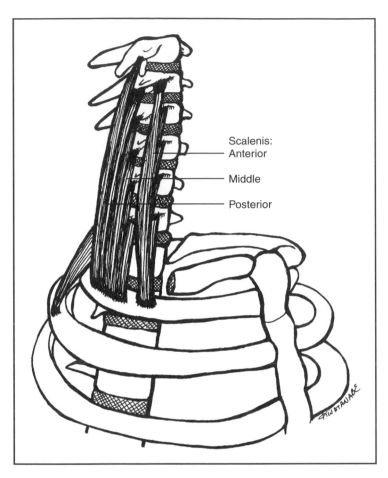

The anterior, medial, and posterior scalenus muscles are shown. The anterior scalenus arises from the anterior tubercles of the transverse processes of C_3 through C_6 and inserts into the superior and inner aspects of the first rib. The medial scalenus arises from the posterior tubercle of the transverse processes of C_2 through C_7 and inserts into the superior aspect of the first rib posterior to the anterior scalenus. The posterior scalenus arises from the posterior tubercles of the transverse processes of C_5, C_6, and C_7 and inserts into the outer surface of the second rib. Fibers of the posterior scalenus may blend with those of the middle scalenus.[1]

Figure 10-2A: Scaleni muscles (anterior-lateral view).

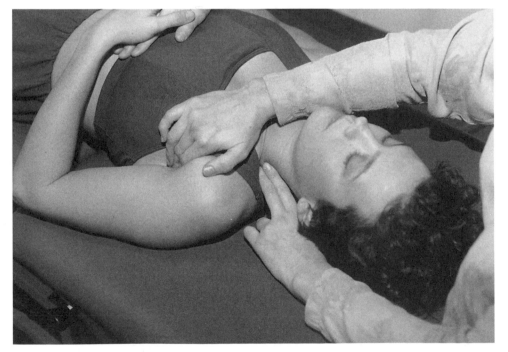

The patient is supine. The therapist sits at the head of the table. The neck is taken into a side-bending movement toward the involved side and can be left positioned there. One hand palpates the involved fibers as the other hand takes the first and second ribs into elevation. If necessary, add neck flexion to isolate the anterior and middle fibers, by placing the head on towel or pillow. Decrease the side bending to a more neutral position if bilateral involvement is noted.

Figure 10-2B: Scalenes release.

The trapezius muscle was discussed in Chapter 9. Its origination and insertion points are shown in Figure 9-7A.

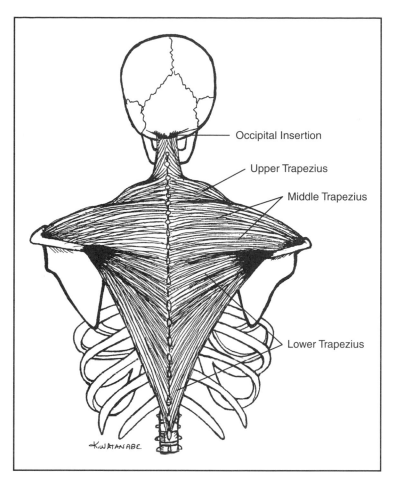

Figure 10-3A: Trapezius muscle (posterior view).

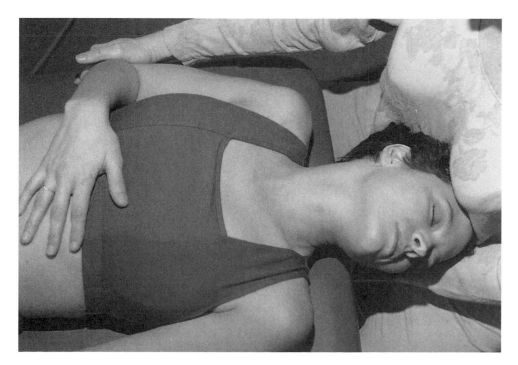

Figure 10-3B: Upper trapezius release.

The patient is supine. The therapist sits at the head of the table. Elevate the scapula by taking the shoulder or scapula superior and medial toward the ear. Rotate the neck to the opposite side, extend and side bend the neck to the same side. The hand that supports the neck can also palpate the involved fibers or position the arm for scapular elevation and have a free hand for palpation. The therapist can fine tune the release through either the neck or shoulder. If necessary, take the head off the table to increase the extension component of the release (shown). Have the patient slide up the table while the therapist supports the neck in the release position. After the release, support the neck as the patient slowly slides back down on the table.

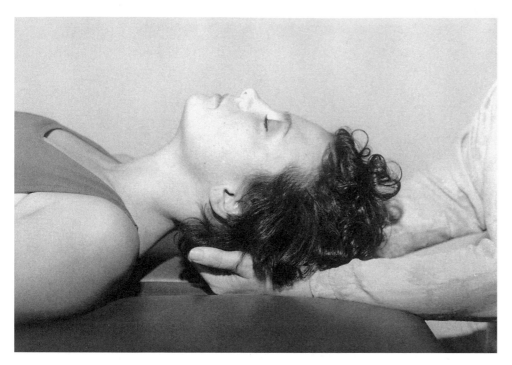

Figure 10-3C: Occipital insertion release of the upper trapezius.

The patient is supine. The therapist sits at the head of the table. With a bilateral handhold of the occiput in the palms of hands, take the neck into extension at the upper cervical area by taking the occiput inferior. Fingertips reach down to the mid neck and traction fibers of the upper trapezius toward the external occipital protuberance. This will slacken the upper fibers. Fine tune the release with both hands, following any rotation or strain pattern present. Certain cranial restrictions will inhibit the ability to mobilize the occiput and make this release difficult or impossible to carry out.

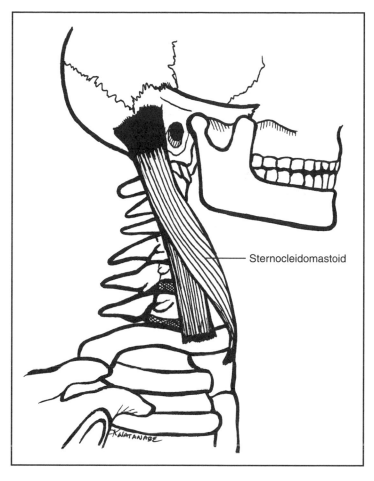

Figure 10-4A: Sternocleidomastoid muscle (lateral view).

The sternocleidomastoid arises from two heads: the medial head originates from the superior anterior surface of the manubrium of the sternum while the lateral head originates from the superior and anterior surfaces of the middle third of the clavicle. The insertion is into the lateral surface of the mastoid process of the temporal bone with a thin aponeurosis inserting into the superior nuchal line of the occiput.[1]

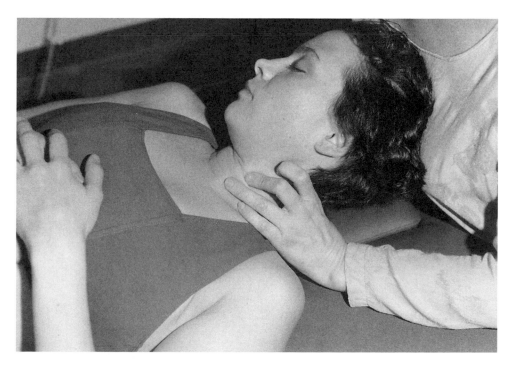

Figure 10-4B: Sternocleidomastoid release.

The patient is supine. The therapist sits at the head of the table. Take the neck into flexion with rotation to the opposite side and side bending to same side. One hand can support the head in this position while the other hand palpates. If necessary, sacrifice the palpating hand to elevate the clavicle.

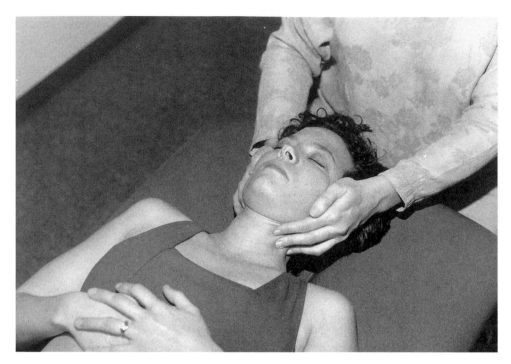

Figure 10-4C: Bilateral sternocleidomastoid release.

The patient is supine. The therapist sits at the head of the table. Release the mastoid insertion by a bilateral handhold of palms on the temporal bones (avoid pressure). Fingertips reach to the mid neck to traction the muscle belly of the sternocleidomastoid superior toward the mastoid. Any rotational strain patterns in neck or temporal bones can be followed more easily with a bilateral hold position. This is an excellent release for temporal mandibular dysfunction. Treatment of this muscle may be helpful with occipital-mastoid cranial restrictions.

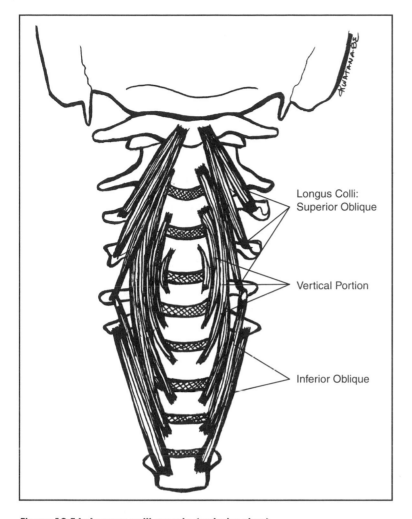

Figure 10-5A: Longus colli muscle (anterior view).

The longus colli consists of three parts: the superior and inferior oblique and the vertical portions. The superior oblique portion arises from the anterior tubercles of the transverse processes of C_3, C_4, and C_5 and ascends to insert on the anterior arch of the atlas. The inferior oblique portion arises from the anterior surface of the bodies of T_1 and T_2 (T_3) and ascends to insert into the anterior tubercles of the transverse processes of C_5 and C_6. The vertical portion arises from the anterior surface of the bodies of C_4 through T_3 and inserts into the anterior surface of the bodies of C_2, C_3, and C_4.[1]

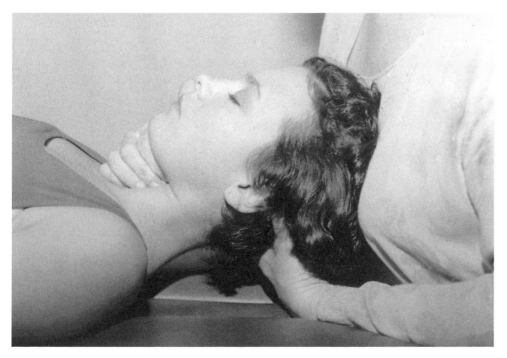

Figure 10-5B: Longus colli release.

The patient is supine. The therapist sits at the head of the table. Move the superficial structures of larynx and trachea to the side. The muscle lies anterior to sternocleidomastoid muscle. Use layer palpation to find the deep fibers, which lie anterior to the bodies of the cervical and upper thoracic vertebrae. Avoid any pressure on the carotid artery, especially if carotid artery disease is present or suspected. Skip the palpation step if you are hesitant about contraindications in this vulnerable region. To release the longus colli, take the neck into a forward flexion with side bending toward same side and rotation, as necessary, to fine tune the release.

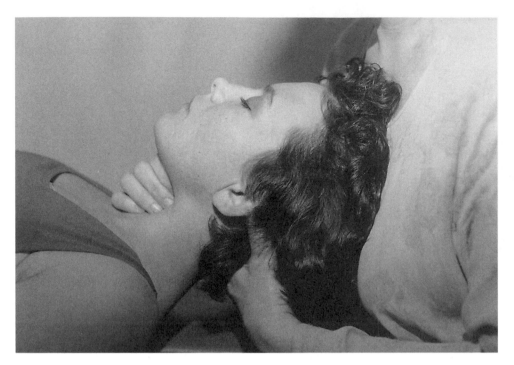

Figure 10-5C: Longus colli release with a forward head posture.

This muscle frequently is involved in whiplash injuries. It can maintain a forward head position if chronically shortened. If the patient presents a forward head posture, it may be necessary to recreate it during the release. In this case, first recreate the patient's pattern, then take the neck into flexion (side bending and rotation) from that position. Use slight compression to recreate the chronic shortening of muscle fibers sometimes found.

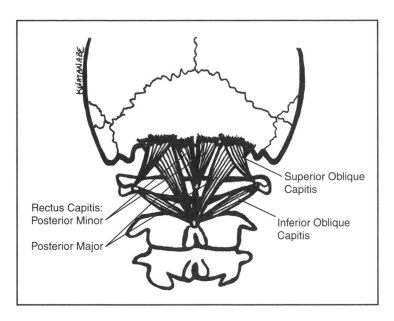

Figure 10-6A: Suboccipital muscles (posterior view).

Rectus Capitis:
Posterior Minor

Posterior Major

Superior Oblique
Capitis

Inferior Oblique
Capitis

The suboccipitals include the obliqus capitis superior and inferior and the rectus capitis posterior major and minor. The obliqus capitis superior arises from the C_1 (atlas) transverse process and inserts into the occiput between the superior and inferior nuchal lines. The rectus capitis posterior major arises from the spinous process of C_2 and inserts into the occiput on the lateral aspect of the inferior nuchal line. The rectus capitis posterior minor arises from the posterior arch of the atlas and inserts into the occiput on the medial aspect of the inferior nuchal line. The obliqus capitus inferior arises from the spinous process of C_2 (axis) and inserts into the transverse process of C_1.[1]

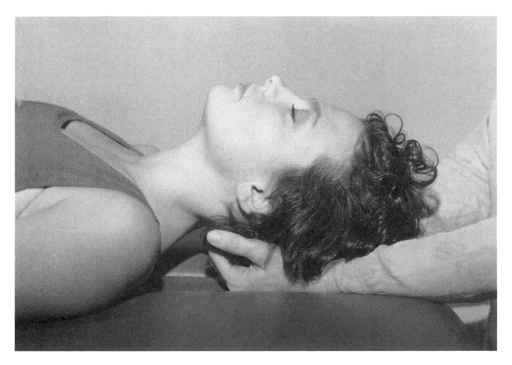

Figure 10-6B: Suboccipital general release.

The patient is supine. The therapist sits at the head of the table. For a general release of the suboccipitals (rectus capitis posterior major and minor and the superior oblique muscles), take the neck into an upper cervical extension and rotate the head to the same side. Take the occiput insertion inferior as you traction C_1 and C_2 in a superior direction. Focus primarily on the extension component and follow any rotational strain patterns present.

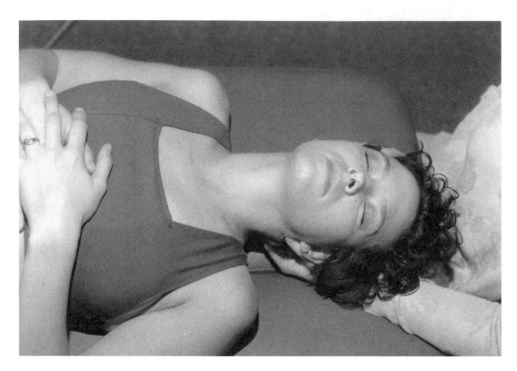

Figure 10-6C: Obliqus capitis inferior release.

The patient is supine. The therapist sits at the head of the table. The neck rotates toward the same side, when you release the obliqus capitis inferior by rotating the atlas on the axis. Stabilize the C_2 spinous process with one hand and palpate as you rotate the transverse process of C_1 toward the side you are releasing.

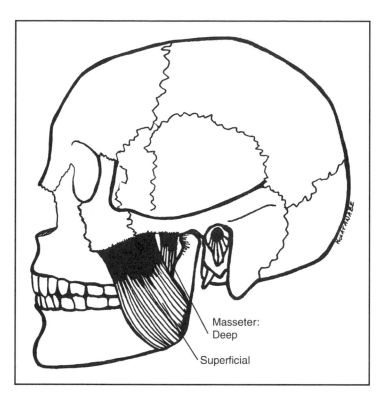

Figure 10-7A: Masseter muscle (lateral view).

The masseter muscle, which elevates the jaw, has a much larger superficial portion and a smaller deep portion. The anterior superficial fibers contribute to the protrusion, while the deep fibers contribute to retraction of the mandible. The superficial portion arises from the anterior inferior aspect of the zygomatic arch and the maxilla (zygomatic process) and inserts into mandible at the angle and the inferior half of the ramus on the lateral surface. The deep portion arises from the posterior, medial, and inferior aspects of the zygomatic arch and inserts into the superior half of the ramus of the mandible on the coronoid process.[1]

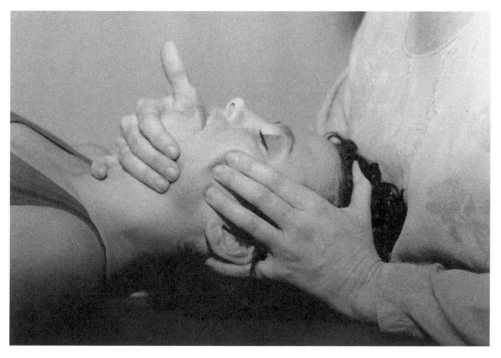

Figure 10-7B: Masseter release.

The patient is supine. The therapist sits at the head of the table. One hand stabilizes the origin through the zygoma if the patient can tolerate this, or a frontal or parietal hold if unable to tolerate. The other hand takes the involved side into elevation with a slight lateral glide to the same side to line up fibers inserting into mandible with the zygomatic origin. Do a bilateral release by taking the mandible into elevation while stabilizing the zygomatic arches with a bilateral handhold (not shown). Follow any rotational strain patterns present. Do not jam the condyle into the temporal fossa with this or the temporalis release, as very little movement is available (millimeters) at the temporal mandibular joint (TMJ).

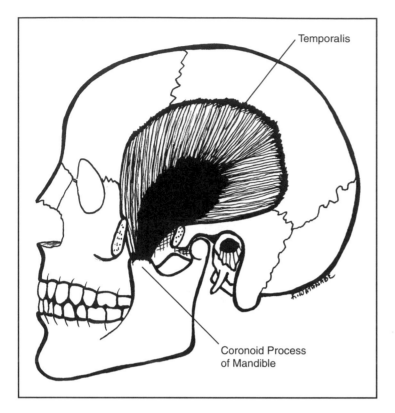

Figure 10-8A: Temporalis muscle (lateral view).

Origin of the temporalis is very broad, primarily from the parietal bone but also from the frontal, temporal, and sphenoid bones. The temporalis arises from the entire temporal fossa and also has an extensive fascial origin. The tendon passes under the zygomatic arch, but does not attach there. It inserts into the mandible at the coronoid process and the anterior border of the ramus.[1]

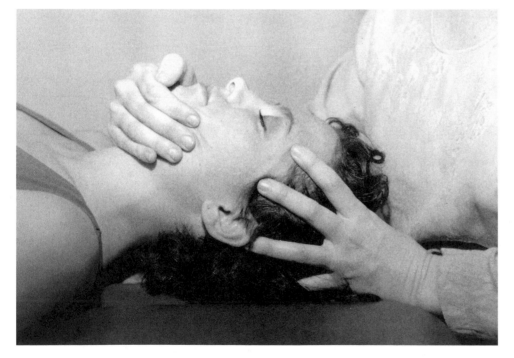

Figure 10-8B: Temporalis release.

The patient is supine. The therapist sits at the head of the table. Take the parietal bone inferior and anterior with one hand while the other hand takes the mandible into elevation with retraction. Palpate the temporalis insertion intraorally on the coronoid process of the mandible before, during, or after the release, if desired. If bilateral involvement is noted, first palpate and check for ease and bind in the temporalis to assess which release to do first. All intraoral releases are done with a gloved hand.

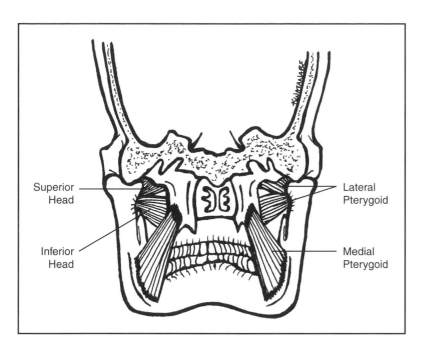

Figure 10-9A: Medial and lateral pterygoid muscles (posterior view).

The medial (internal) pterygoid arises from the pterygoid plate of the sphenoid bone, the palatine bone, and the tuberosity of the maxillae, by two slips. It inserts into the angle and inferior half of the ramus of the mandible on the medial surface. The lateral (external) pterygoid arises from two heads. The superior head originates from the sphenoid bone on the inferior lateral aspect of the greater wing and the infratemporal crest, while the inferior head originates from the lateral pterygoid plate of the sphenoid. Both heads converge and insert into the neck of the condyle of the mandible.[1]

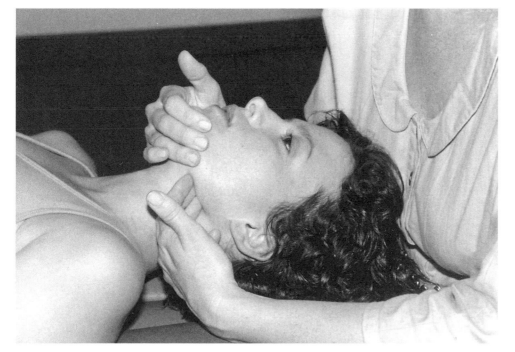

Figure 10-9B: Medial pterygoid release.

The patient is supine. The therapist sits at the head of the table toward the uninvolved side. The medial pterygoid can be palpated either externally on its insertion under the angle and ramus of the mandible or intraorally on its origin at the medial pterygoid plate. One hand can palpate externally and take the mandible into elevation, protrusion, and lateral glide to the opposite side.

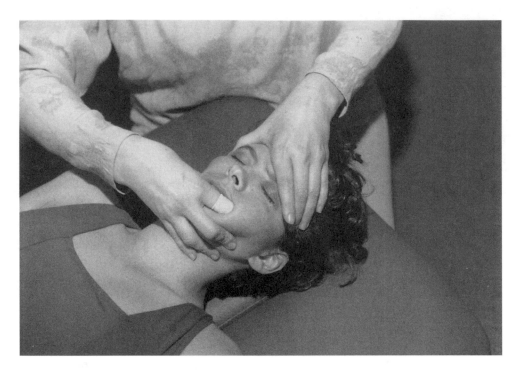

Figure 10-9C: Lateral pterygoid release.

The patient is supine. The therapist sits at the head of the table toward the uninvolved side. Use the index finger of your lower hand to palpate the lateral pterygoid intraorally on the lateral pterygoid plate of the sphenoid. The same palpating hand then takes the mandible into a slight depression, protrusion, and lateral glide away from side you are releasing. The other hand can take the sphenoid anterior and inferior and fine tune the release, with a bilateral hold on the greater wings.

Reference

1. Gray H; edited by Goss CM. *Gray's Anatomy of the Human Body*. 29th ed. Philadelphia: Lea and Febiger, 1973.

11

Paraspinal Muscular Application

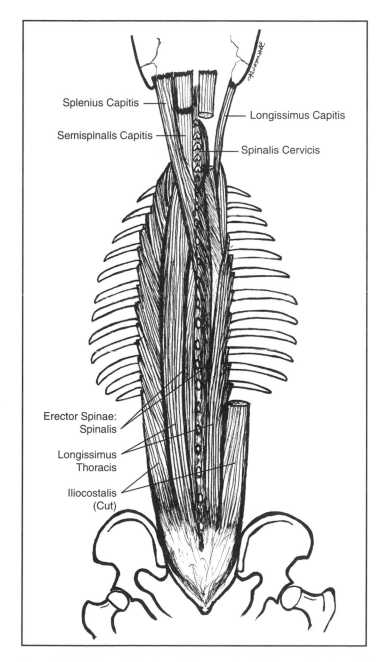

Splenius Capitis

Semispinalis Capitis

Erector Spinae:
Spinalis

Longissimus
Thoracis

Iliocostalis
(Cut)

Longissimus Capitis

Spinalis Cervicis

Figure 11-1A: Iliocostalis, longissimus, and spinalis muscles (posterior view).

The erector spinae muscle group arises from the sacrum, the spinous processes of T_{12} through L_5, the supraspinal ligament, and the iliac crest (posterior inner lip) and blends with fibers from the gluteus maximus, sacrotuberous, and posterior sacroiliac ligaments. As this muscle group ascends alongside the vertebral column, it splits into three columns: the lateral muscle group is the iliocostalis, the intermediate group is the longissimus, and the medial group is the spinalis. Each of these three narrow bands of muscle divides further into three muscles, all with thoracic and cervical sections. The iliocostalis has a lumbar component, while the longissimus and spinalis have a capitis component that attaches to the cranium. The iliocostalis and longissimus groups arise and insert into the ribs and transverse processes in their respective region, while the spinalis group arises and inserts on spinous processes. The function of all these muscles is to extend the spine or neck and side bend toward the same side.[1]

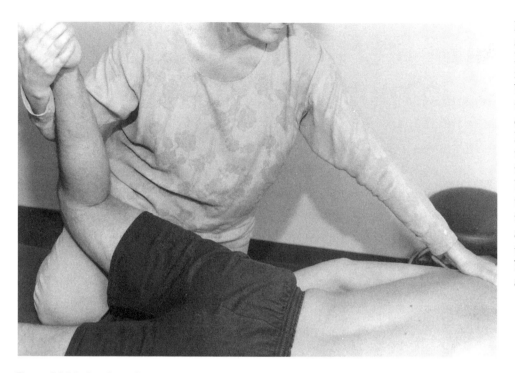

Figure 11-1B: Erector spinae general release.

Position the patient prone. The therapist stands on the involved side. Position the trunk and upper body in extension, either with pillows or by raising the head of table. Take the hip on the involved side into extension or position there with pillows. The trunk is side bent toward the involved side with the head turned toward the involved side. Do a general release by approximation of the erector spinae through the shoulder girdle depression and a superior lift of the ilium, maintaining and increasing the side bending and extension components as necessary.

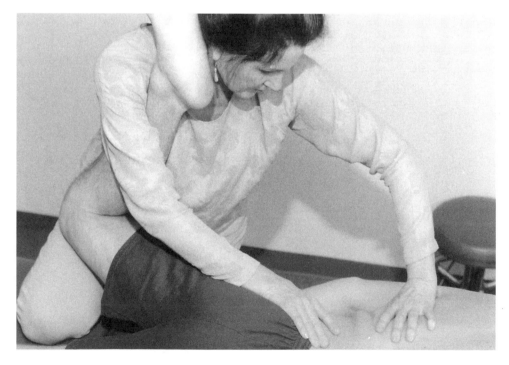

Figure 11-1C: Mid-muscle-group erector spinae release.

Position the patient prone. The therapist stands on the involved side. Extend the spine through elevation of the trunk and hip extension, as described for Figure 11-1B. Locate the area of greatest restriction in the paraspinal muscles through palpation and motion testing of bind and ease. With one hand on either side of involved region, do a mid-muscle release by approximating specifically above and below the area of most involvement. The releases shown are for the lumbar and thoracic region. The superficial paraspinals in the cervical region are released by extension with side bending to the same side (not shown).

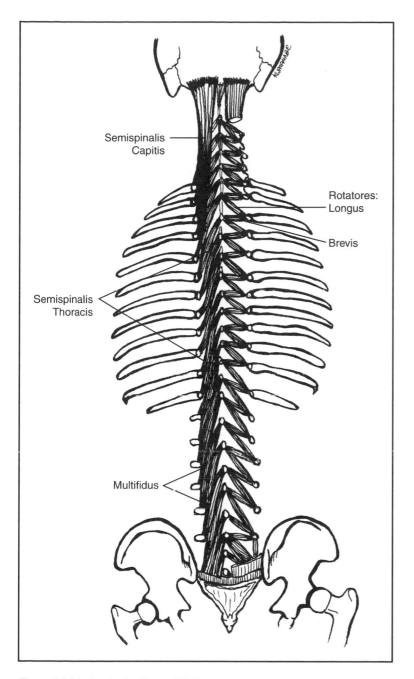

Figure 11-2A: Semispinalis, multifidi, and rotatores muscles (posterior view).

The deep paraspinals, which involve rotation of the spine to the opposite side, include the semispinalis (thoracis and capitis), multifidi, and rotatores (longus and brevis). The multifidi and rotatores are a series of many small muscles that extend the entire length of the vertebral column, from the sacrum to the axis. These muscles originate from the transverse processes and insert onto the spinous process of the vertebrae one to four levels above it. The primary function of all these muscles is to extend and rotate the spine or neck to the opposite side.[1]

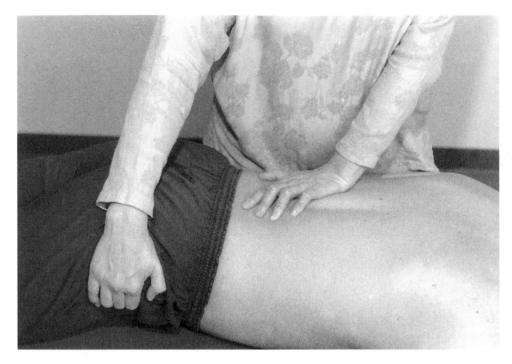

Figure 11-2B: Ilium lift for deep paraspinals release.

The patient is prone. The therapist stands opposite the involved side. Elevate the trunk by raising the head of the table or placing the patient on pillows to create the extension component. To create the rotational component in this release, use the heel of one hand to block the spine at the involved spinous process and the fingertips to palpate the involved area. To address the lumbar and lower thoracic region, an ilium lift is used.

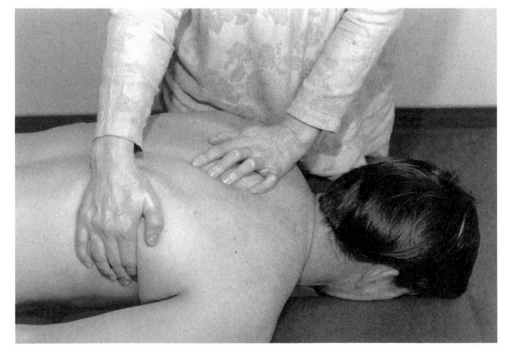

Figure 11-2C: Rib lift for deep paraspinals release.

The patient is prone. The therapist stands opposite the involved side. Elevate the trunk by raising the head of the table or position on pillows to create extension. Block at the spinous process with one hand, while the other hand uses a rib lift to create the rotational component to release the thoracic region. Release the deep paraspinals in the cervical spine by extension with rotation to the opposite side (not shown). If more extension of the neck is required, support the patient with his or her head off the table, as shown in the upper trapezius release (see Figure 10-3B).

Reference

1. Gray H; Goss CM, ed. *Gray's Anatomy of the Human Body.* 29th ed. Philadelphia: Lea and Febiger, 1973.

12

Introduction to Joint Application

Joint Mobilization

The joint application of Positional Release presented in this book presumes that the therapist has a certain basic level knowledge of joint mobilization principles and procedures. A few of Maitland's peripheral and vertebral manipulation principles and procedures will be reviewed here, but further study of these or other books on mobilization is recommended if you have had no previous mobilization experience.[1,2]

Maitland divides passive movements into two groups, those that can be performed actively are called *physiological movements* and those that can be produced only passively are called *accessory movements*. During an objective examination of a joint, active and passive physiological movements and accessory movements of the joint in a neutral position or at the limit of the physiological range are assessed. The passive movements available and other considerations specific to each joint may require further study.[1,2]

Grades of movement describe the amplitude and part of range of movement used in evaluation and treatment. In this book, only Grades I, II, and III are recommended and will be considered. Maitland defined these as, "Grade I: Small amplitude movement performed at the beginning of the range. Grade II: Large amplitude movement performed within the range but not reaching the limit of the range. Grade III: Large amplitude movement performed up to the limit of the range."[1,2] Assessment of the amount of friction or resistance present through the full range of motion or quality of movement as well as the feel of the end range of motion are important observations.

It is easy to apply the indirect principles of Positional Release to known mobilization procedures. Remember that the releases presented here can be adapted to most mobilization procedures. If you are more comfortable or familiar with other mobilization techniques than those shown, please use them.

Application of Joint Mobilization Procedures

A simplification of the complexity of specific joint mobilization techniques is necessary for the Positional Release application presented herein. Remember that skill development in these specific joint mobilization procedures is recommended, as it will greatly increase your effectiveness in indirect treatment techniques. Learning the normal accessory movements at each joint will fine tune your skill base and help you ascertain abnormalities and dysfunction with more ease. It also will help you go into a release with more depth, as you begin to test for more subtle movement possibilities and fine tune with more accuracy. If you stay within the guidelines of movement away from pain and into ease of motion, you most likely will do no harm to a patient using an indirect technique, as compared to the advanced skill base needed to perform a Grade IV or end range mobilization procedure.[1,2]

Assessment of the physiological and accessory joint movement at a target joint is necessary to determine the preferred direction of motion for the release hold. A gentle oscillatory type movement (Grades I, II, and III) is used to assess joint play through the full amplitude of available pain-free range of motion at the joint being assessed. Assessing the end range of the joint in each direction of the range in question is required. Once you determine ease of motion in a certain direction, you will be able to proceed with the release by going away from the restriction or barrier.

Initially, examination and treatment usually are done from a neutral resting position of the joint, but remember that assessment and treatment can be repeated from any point in the physiologic range of motion, based on need. Sometimes a bias of physiological motion is needed in treatment. Again, getting information about the mechanism of injury is important. For example, if a person's wrist was extended while breaking a fall, then it would be important to use a wrist extension bias during treatment. Testing and treatment of joint play would be done both in neutral and with wrist extension in this instance, as the joint restrictions and release positions are different with and without the bias.

The joint releases presented usually start from an assessment of anterior-posterior joint motion. Then other accessory motions are tested including medial-lateral (abduction-adduction), longitudinal compression or distraction, and rotation right and left. Often these motions are done in combination or "stacked" successively to obtain the optimal release position. At times, it may be necessary to repeat or focus on a single accessory motion in isolation to get optimal results. A single motion also may be more appropriate if an isometric is to be used following the release.

Mobilization usually involves stabilization with one hand and assessment of joint mobility with the other hand. The following generalizations regarding the stabilizing and assessing hand may be useful in learning the release techniques. With peripheral joint mobilization techniques, stabilization usually is proximal and mobilization is distal. If a lateral or side-by-side mobilization is to be done, such as with the metatarsal bones, assess motion of the most involved bone and stabilize the adjacent bone that feels most directly involved or related to the restriction. Stabilization of the larger bone while mobilizing the smaller bone also is recommended during the joint assessment, such as with the proximal or distal tibia-fibula joint.

Comfort and relaxation of the patient are important during the testing and release process. Support the patient in a neutral resting position and use pillows or towel rolls to fill in the spaces not in contact with the table (such as under the knees), as necessary, to obtain an optimal relaxation response. Also it is important to keep both hands as relaxed as possible and to use a comfortable broad surface contact of hands and fingers during the assessment and release process.

Joint Releases

Therapists sometimes have difficulty with the concept of joint releases because joints do not have the same proprioceptive components (such as muscle spindles) as muscles, since the neuromuscular mechanism is thought to be responsible for the release phenomenon. The separation of the body into muscles and joints is an artificial delineation, useful for teaching and learning more than actual treatment. While it is entirely possible to isolate a muscle, joint, or ligament as a treatment focus, it is not possible to eliminate the influence or relationship of surrounding tissues and structures to that target tissue. Anytime you treat a joint there must be consideration of the muscular elements around that joint. Perhaps, joint releases are primarily achieved by affecting the muscular component through afferent reduction. Keep in mind that the origins of this work are osteopathic and, therefore, most literature on indirect work describes joint not muscular applications.

After assessing joint motion just described, you can determine the preferred direction away from the restrictive barrier into ease of motion. Take the joint away from the barrier or restriction into a pain-free position, where all the tissues around the joint are relaxed. This basic release position can be fine-tuned through stacking other accessory motions or adding the rotational and compression or distraction components to the release.

Hold the release position for 60–90 seconds or until you palpate for a release, as discussed earlier. Take the patient slowly and passively out of the release position with support, so he or she does not actively engage the surrounding muscles. Reassess joint motion by repeating your mobilization process again. Sometimes, certain restrictions will clear out easily, which allows other restrictions to be more evident. If necessary, repeat the release or modify it to more accurately address the specific joint restrictions present. Isometrics can be used quite successfully with all joint releases as with muscular releases (see Chapter 17). The same treatment considerations discussed in Chapter 7 for muscular application apply to joint applications.

Summary

1. Assess physiological and accessory joint motion.
2. Determine the preferred direction of motion away from the restrictive barrier.
3. Fine-tune the release position.
4. Hold the release for 60–90 seconds, or until you palpate the release.
5. Perform an isometric out of the release position, if necessary.
6. Take the patient slowly and passively out of the release position with support.
7. Reassess physiological and accessory joint motion.
8. Repeat release procedure or modify to more specifically address joint restrictions.

References

1. Maitland GD. *Peripheral Manipulation*. 2nd ed. London: Butterworths; 1977.
2. Maitland GD. *Vertebral Manipulation*. 4th ed. London: Butterworths; 1977.

13

Pelvis and Lower Extremity Joint Application

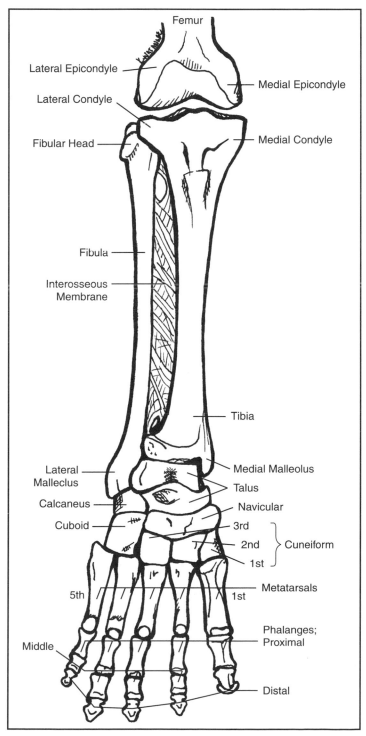

Figure 13-1: Foot, ankle, and knee joints (anterior view).

Femur

Lateral Epicondyle

Medial Epicondyle

Lateral Condyle

Medial Condyle

Fibular Head

Fibula

Interosseous Membrane

Tibia

Medial Malleolus

Lateral Malleclus

Talus

Calcaneus

Navicular

Cuboid

3rd

2nd   Cuneiform

1st

Metatarsals

5th   1st

Phalanges; Proximal

Middle

Distal

Figure 13-1 shows the bones of the ankle, tibia, fibula, interosseous membrane, and knee joint (the patella is not shown). This drawing provides an anatomical reference for releases shown in Figures 13-2 through 13-14.

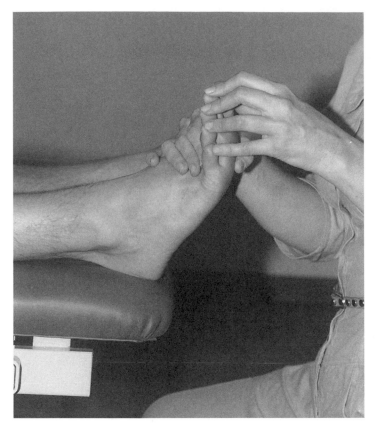

Figure 13-2: Metatarsal phalange release.

The patient is supine. The therapist sits at the foot of the table. Release dropped metatarsal heads by taking toes into dorsiflexion to exaggerate their unique foot posture. The other hand palpates around the anterior and posterior aspect of all metatarsal phalange joints of the involved foot. Add pronation (or supination) as needed to fine tune the release.

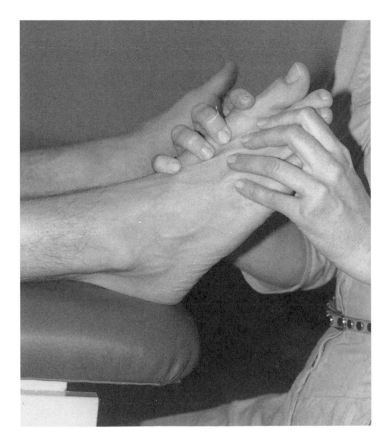

Figure 13-3: Intermetatarsal release.

The patient is supine. The therapist sits at the foot of the table. Assess the joint motion between metatarsal bones and determine any inferior-superior restrictions. Follow the restrictions found by exaggeration. Use the rotational component to fine tune the release.

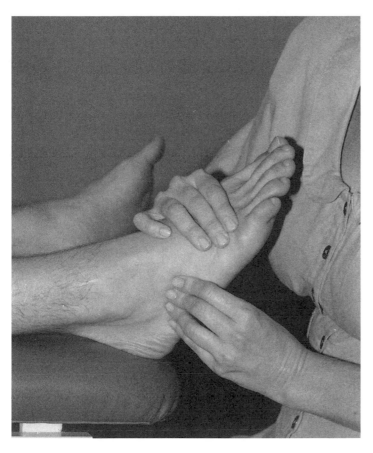

The patient is supine. The therapist sits at the foot of table. Assess the anterior-posterior motion of the cuboid to see if it is dropped (the typical pattern) or elevated. Exaggerate the position of the cuboid and add rotation (usually lateral) through the fourth and fifth metatarsals to fine tune the release. With a dropped cuboid, you can also add compression through the calcaneous toward the cuboid to facilitate the release as needed (not shown).

Figure 13-4: Cuboid release.

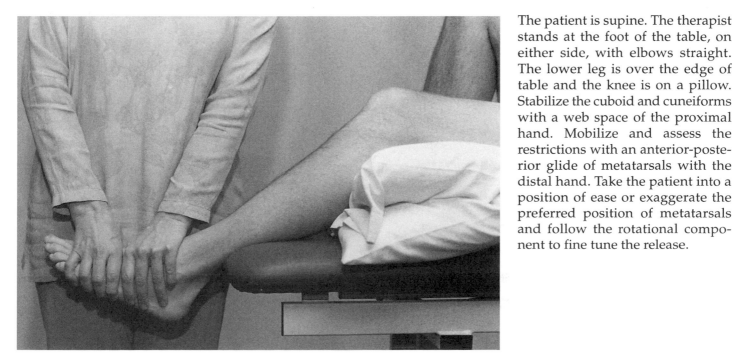

The patient is supine. The therapist stands at the foot of the table, on either side, with elbows straight. The lower leg is over the edge of table and the knee is on a pillow. Stabilize the cuboid and cuneiforms with a web space of the proximal hand. Mobilize and assess the restrictions with an anterior-posterior glide of metatarsals with the distal hand. Take the patient into a position of ease or exaggerate the preferred position of metatarsals and follow the rotational component to fine tune the release.

Figure 13-5: Tarsometatarsal release.

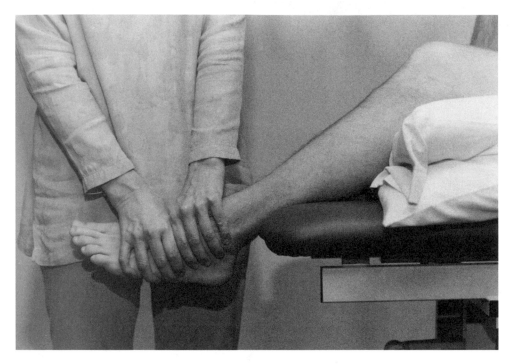

The patient is supine. The therapist stands at the foot of the table, on either side, with elbows straight. Stabilize the talus and calcaneous with the proximal hand and mobilize the navicular and cuboid with distal hand in an anterior-posterior glide. Assess restrictions and follow into the position of ease. Follow the rotational component to fine tune the release.

Figure 13-6: Talonavicular-calcanocuboid release.

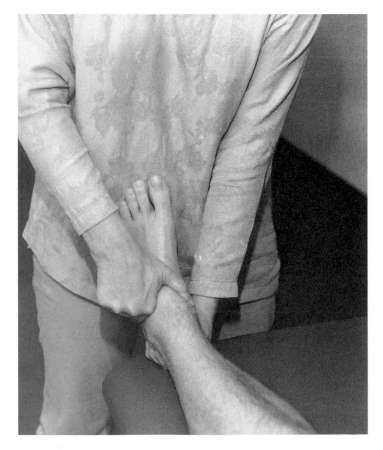

The patient is supine. The therapist stands at the foot of the table. One hand stabilizes the calcaneous, while the index and thumb of the other hand motion assesses the talus in an anterior-medial and posterior-lateral combined movement. Take the patient into ease of motion and again add the rotational component to fine tune the release.

Figure 13-7: Subtalar joint-talocalcaneal release.

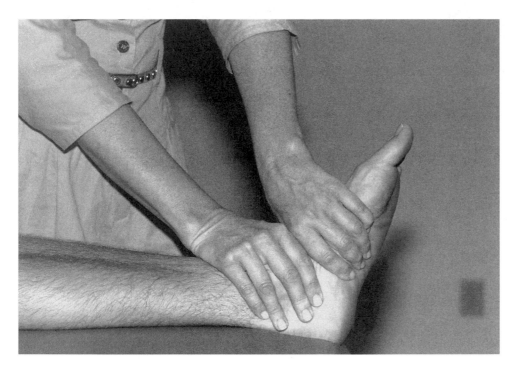

Figure 13-8: Tibia-talus override.

The patient is supine. The therapist stands at the end of the table on the side of the involved foot. The tibia has overridden the talus, with a sudden stop as in running. The junction will be point tender and a "step" will be present when compared to the other side. One hand does an anterior glide of the tibia as the other hand does a posterior glide of the talus to release.[1]

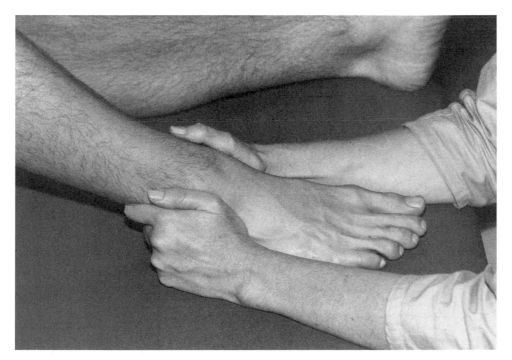

Figure 13-9: Inferior tibia-fibula release.

The patient is supine. The therapist sits at the foot of the table. Flex the involved leg with the foot resting on the table. One hand stabilizes tibia at the medial malleolus, while the other hand motion tests the fibula in an anterior-lateral and posterior-medial combined motion through the lateral malleolus. Both hands should use a broad surface contact between the thumb, which is anterior to the malleolus, and the index finger, which is behind the malleolus, to assure patient comfort during the examination and release.

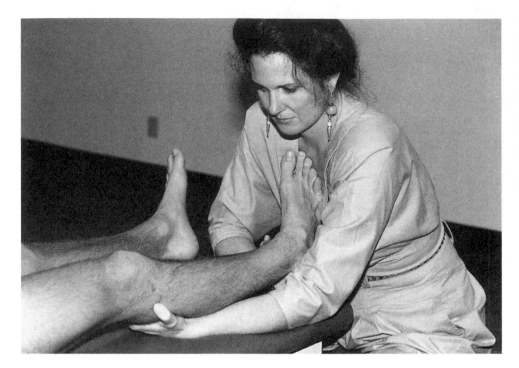

The patient is supine. The therapist sits at the foot of the table. One hand holds the tibia and fibula proximally around the superior tibia-fibula joint, and one hand holds the bones distally at the inferior tibia-fibula joint. Stabilize proximally and rotate distally to determine any strain patterns present throughout the interosseous membrane. This requires layer palpation to a deep membranous level.

Figure 13-10: Interosseous membrane release.

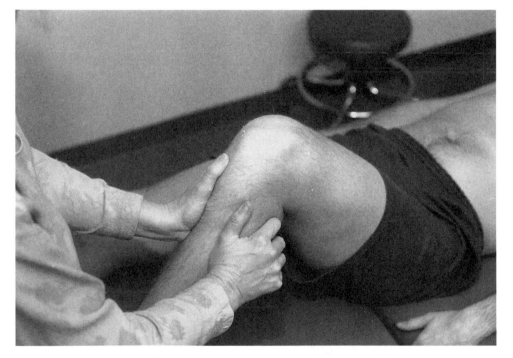

The patient is supine. Flex the leg with the foot resting on the table. The therapist sits on the involved side. One hand stabilizes the tibia as the other hand mobilizes the fibula in an anterior posterior direction. Use broad surface contact between the thumb and index finger for motion assessment and release. Take the patient into a position of ease and follow the rotational component to fine tune the release. Add longitudinal distraction or compression with straight leg, if needed.

Figure 13-11: Superior tibia-fibula release.

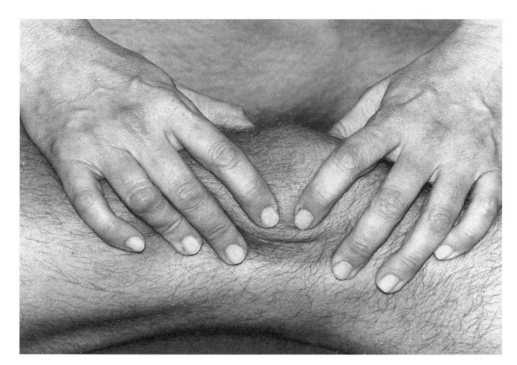

Figure 13-12: Patellar release.

The patient is supine. The therapist stands on the involved side. Assess the motions and take the patient into a position of ease. Check superior-inferior, medial-lateral, medial-lateral tilt, and clockwise-counterclockwise rotation motions to determine preference. You can treat each motion individually or stack motions. With postarthroscopy or other incisions, take the patella toward point-tender areas of scar tissue to release. This release is easy to teach as self-treatment, with the patient's back supported against a wall while in long sitting.

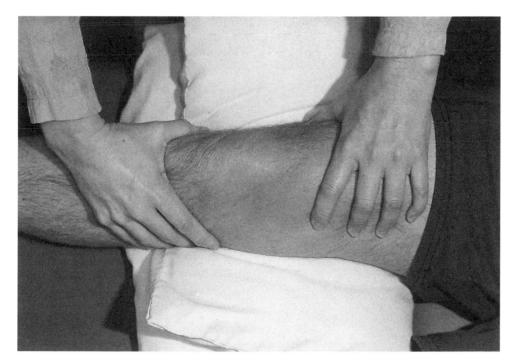

Figure 13-13: Tibia-femoral rotation release.

The patient is supine with the knee bent resting on a pillow. The therapist stands on the involved side. One hand stabilizes the femur while the other hand mobilizes the tibia into medial and lateral rotation. Take tibia into a position of ease for the release with compression or longitudinal distraction to fine tune the release.

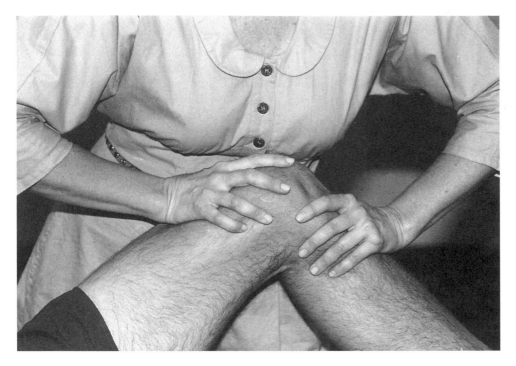

Figure 13-14A: Femur-tibia override.

The patient is supine. The therapist stands on the involved side. First check the passive knee hyperextension with the leg straight and compare it to the other side. This release is indicated if the end feel is hard and the knee is lacking in terminal extension or hyperextension, compared to the other side. For the release, position knee in about 60° (or more) of flexion, with the foot resting on the table. One hand takes the femur anteriorly as the other hand takes the tibia posteriorly to exaggerate the override. This can also be accomplished by placing the practitioner's extended arm under the involved knee and resting it on the opposite femur (not shown). Add a rotational component to fine tune the release as needed.

Complete the release by doing an isometric into a knee extension.[1]

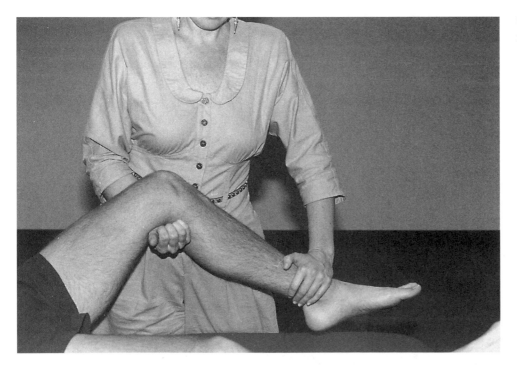

Figure 13-14B: The release is completed by doing an isometric into knee extension.

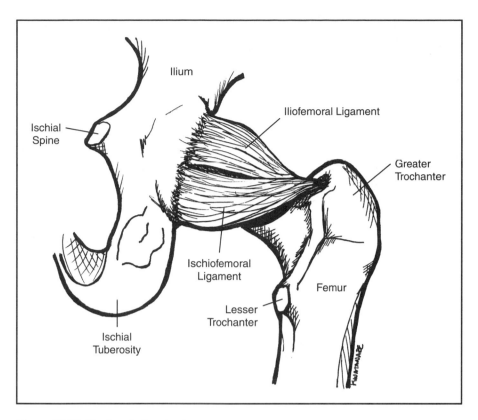

Figure 13-15: Hip (posterior view).

Figure 13-15 shows a posterior view of the hip joint with the ischiofemoral and iliofemoral ligaments. This drawing provides an anatomical reference for releases show in Figures 13-16 through 13-18.

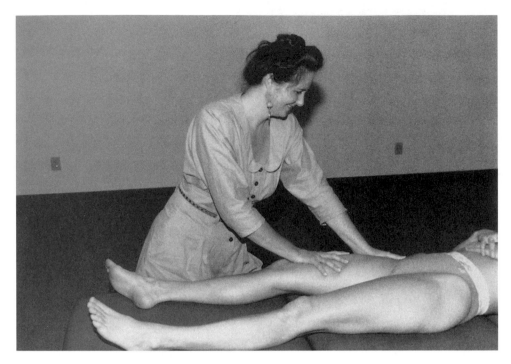

The patient is supine with the leg extended. The therapist stands on the involved side. Both hands are on the femur with full surface contact close to the joint. Assess the preferred rotational motion with deep-layer palpation down to the level of the ligaments. Take the leg into external rotation, which addresses the ischiofemoral ligament.

Figure 13-16: Hip, external rotation release.

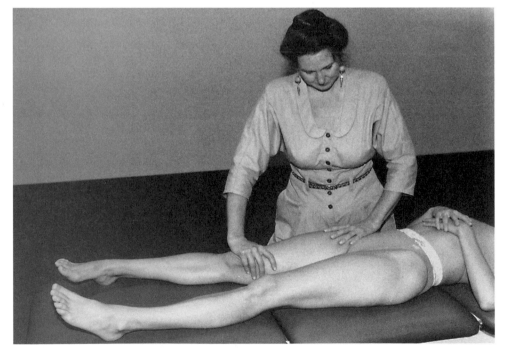

The patient is supine with the leg extended. The therapist stands on the involved side. Both hands are on the femur with full surface contact close to the joint. Assess the preferred rotational motion with deep-layer palpation down to the level of the ligaments. Take the leg into internal rotation, which addresses the iliofemoral ligament.

Figure 13-17: Hip, internal rotation release.

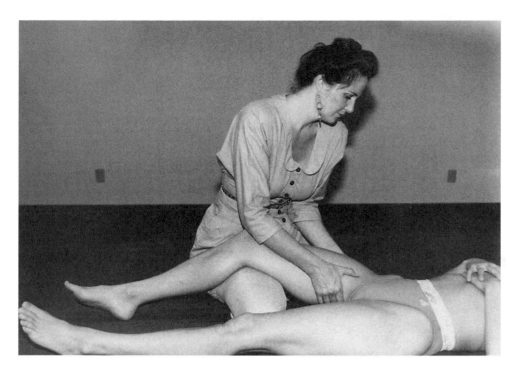

Figure 13-18: Hip mobilization release.

The patient is supine with the hip and knee slightly bent and resting on therapist's leg (or pillow). Hold the hip with a broad surface contact of both hands around the joint, as close to the joint as possible. Assess the following motions: (1) anterior-posterior, (2) medial-lateral, (3) internal-external rotation, and (4) longitudinal distraction-compression. Note any restrictions and follow the patient into a position of ease of motion for the release. Motions can be stacked for a quicker release or done individually, if needed.

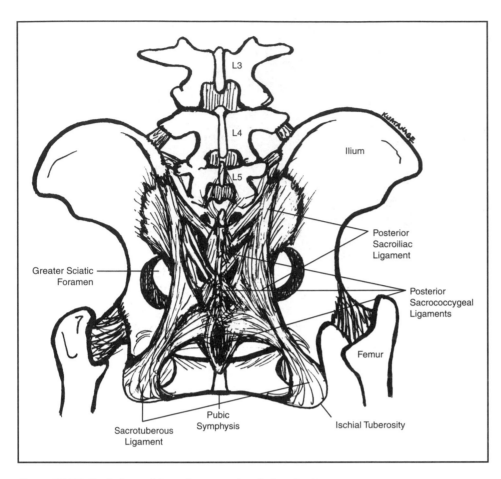

Figure 13-19: Posterior pelvis and sacrum (posterior view).

Figure 13-19 shows the posterior pelvis and sacrum with the sacrotuberous and posterior sacroiliac ligaments. The sacrum is covered posteriorly by ligamentous tissue. This drawing provides an anatomical reference for the releases shown in Figures 13-20 through 13-25.

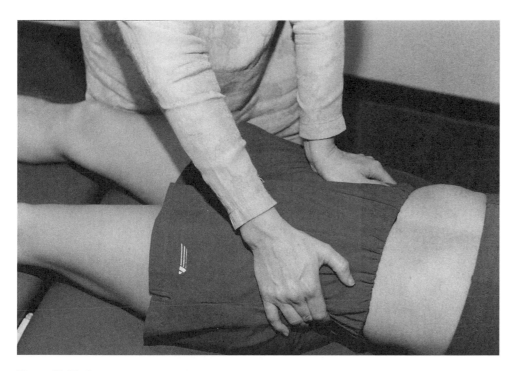

Figure 13-20: General pelvic rotation release.

The examination and release are done with the patient supine. The therapist assesses the anterior-posterior pelvic rotation through motion testing from both sides or kneels over patient for evaluation from a neutral position. The therapist can also assess for upslip, downslip, inflare, and outflare of ilium with motion testing. Other diagnostic tests, such as a standing flexion or squish test, can be used if the therapist is familiar with these evaluation procedures. Check the medial malleolus with the patient supine to assess for long (anterior rotated ilium) or short leg (posterior rotated ilium). If the test results do not agree, go with your motion testing results. For the release, the therapist stands on the side of the posterior-rotated ilium. Take the ilium further into its rotational preference. In addition to the rotational component, follow the ilium in all three planes, recreating any upslip, downslip, inflare, or outflare found. If this general release is not effective in releasing the pattern, follow it with an isometric or see the more specific releases for anterior or posterior rotations, which follow.

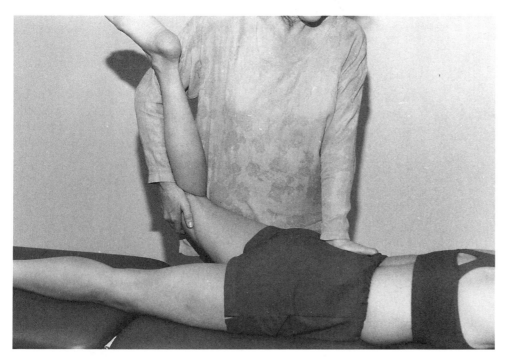

Figure 13-21: Anterior pelvic rotation release.

The patient is prone. The therapist stands on the involved side. Lift the hip into extension with one hand while other hand rotates the ilium anteriorly, with pressure through the heel of hand on the iliac crest. Best results are achieved by creating a force couple around the ilium as described, rather than by resting the hip in extension on a pillow.[1]

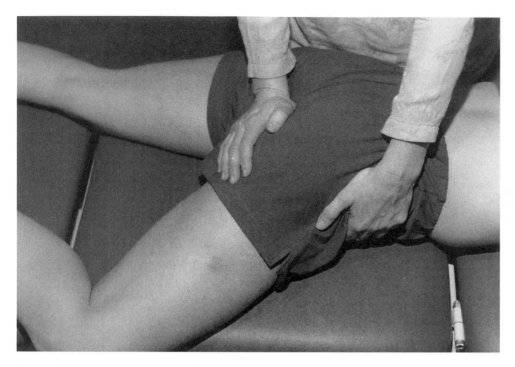

The patient is prone. The therapist stands opposite the involved side. The hip and knee are placed in a flexion, abduction, and external rotation position (frog leg). One hand rotates the ilium posteriorly through an anterior hand hold, as the other hand rotates the ischium anteriorly. Create a force couple around the ilium for best results.[1]

Figure 13-22: Posterior pelvic rotation release.

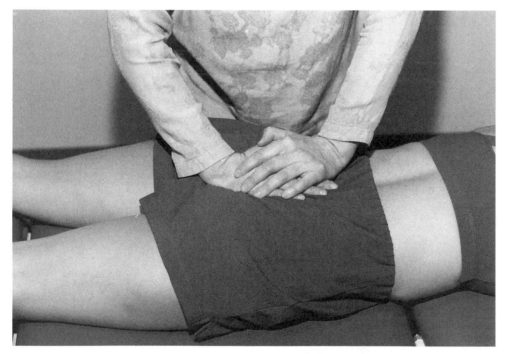

The patient is prone. The therapist stands on either side. Place one palm with full surface contact over the sacrum and other hand atop the first hand. The ligamentous reinforcement around the sacrum is very extensive, so disengage the sacroiliac joints with a downward pressure through both hands. Motion test for flexion-extension, left-right side-bending. and left-right rotation of the sacrum. Recreate the pattern present in all three planes. Motions can be stacked or releases done individually.

Figure 13-23: General sacrum release.

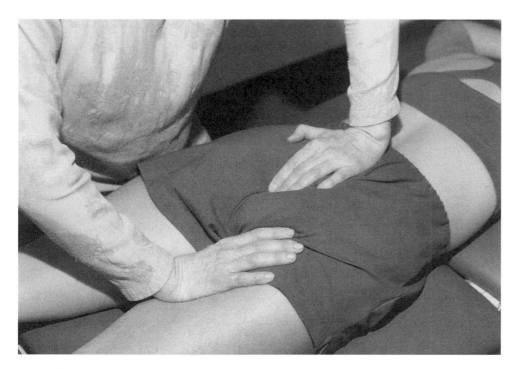

Figure 13-24: Sacrotuberous ligament release.

The patient is prone. The therapist stands opposite the involved side. One hand tractions the sacrum inferior and lateral, as the other hand lifts the ischial tuberosity toward the sacral insertion. This will take the hip into some external rotation, as the hand rotates medially. The sacrotuberous ligament, which attaches to the lower sacrum and coccyx and the ischial tuberosity, often is involved when there is hypermobility at the sacroiliac joint. Remember, this ligament is part of the origin of the gluteus maximus muscle (see Figure 8-5).

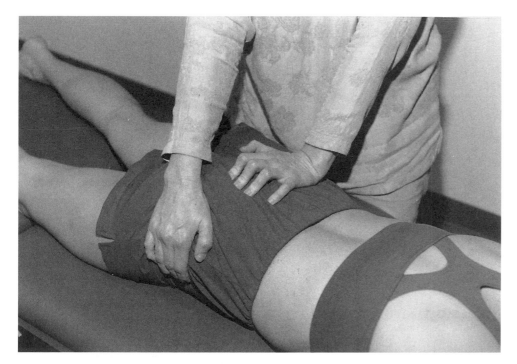

Figure 13-25: Posterior sacroiliac ligament release.

The patient is prone. The therapist stands opposite the involved side. One hand stabilizes the sacrum and palpates as the other hand lifts the ilium posterior and medial. There will be slight variations in the lifts according to which portion of the ligament you are addressing.

Reference

1. Kain K with Berns J. *Ortho-Bionomy®: A Practical Manual.* Berkeley, CA: North Atlantic Books; 1997.

14

Trunk and Upper Extremity Joint Application

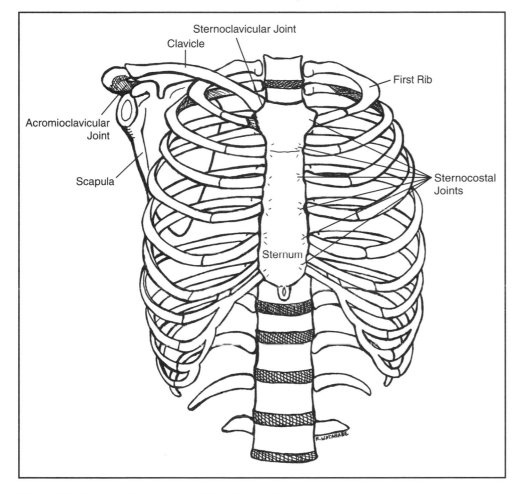

Figure 14-1 shows an anterior view of the thorax including the sternum and ribs. This drawing provides an anatomical reference for the releases shown in Figures 14-2 through 14-6.

Figure 14-1: Thorax—Sternum and rib joints (anterior view).

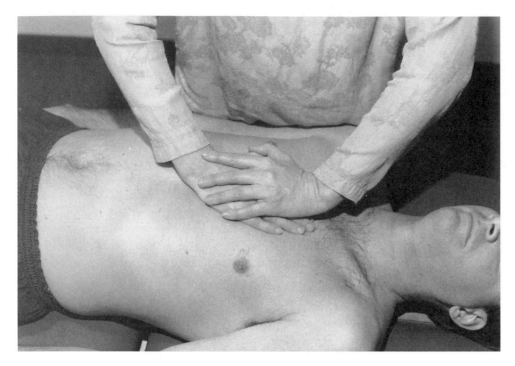

The patient is supine. The therapist stands on either side. Place one palm over the body of the sternum and other hand atop the first. Motion test flexion and extension, side bending right and left, and rotation right and left. Take the sternum into the preferred motions in all three planes or a single plane for release.

Figure 14-2: General sternal release.

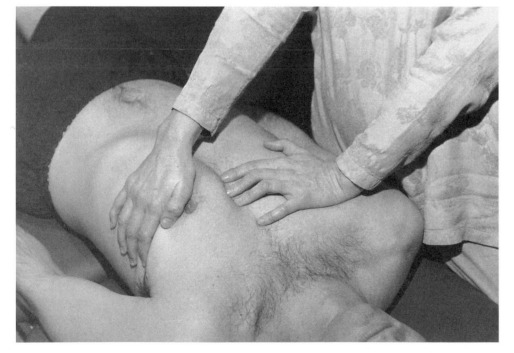

The patient is supine. The therapist stands opposite the involved side. One hand blocks the sternum and palpates the involved sternocostal junction (the area often is slightly raised and point tender). The other hand lifts the involved rib toward the sternum. You can release a single rib or treat several ribs at once.[1]

Figure 14-3: Sternocostal override release.

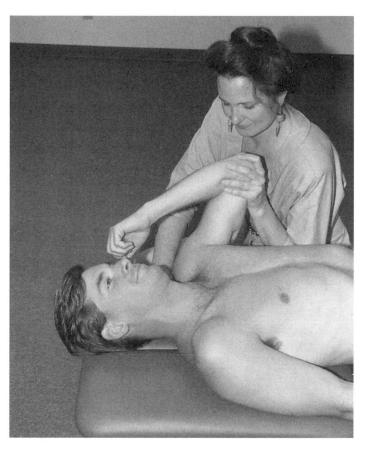

Figure 14-4A: First rib isometric.

The patient is supine. Sit at the head of the table and palpate to determine an elevated first rib. The therapist sits on the involved side and does an isometric preceding the release. Do one of two isometrics: either a shoulder extension from 90° of shoulder flexion (shown) or shoulder adduction from 90° of shoulder abduction (not shown). After isometric contraction, follow the motion through to completion (extension or adduction). The adduction isometric and release can also be modified and done prone (not shown).[1]

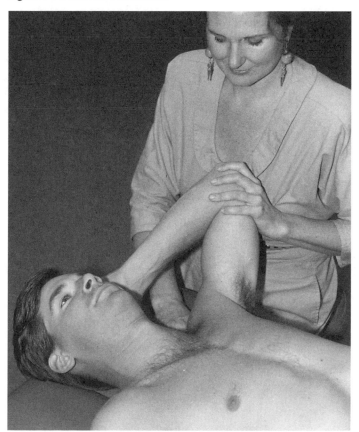

Figure 14-4B: First rib release.

Immediately following the isometric, take the arm into the release position, which generally is found in a hand-to-ear position. Use the rotational component through the elbow to fine tune the release. Palpate the first rib during the entire procedure: isometric, follow-through, and release.[1]

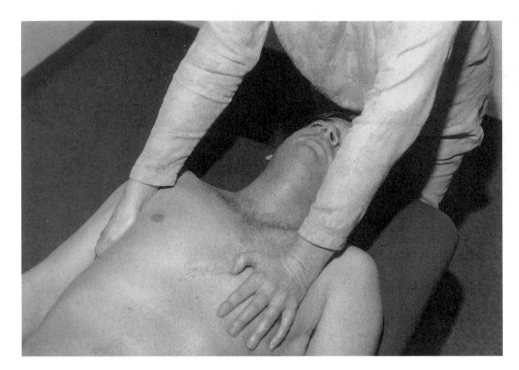

Figure 14-5: Second rib release.

The patient is supine. The therapist stands at the head of the table. Assess the anterior-posterior motion with broad surface contact of the palms on the second ribs. If a posterior rib is found, maintain posterior pressure on it as you lift the opposite side anterior with your hand under the thorax.

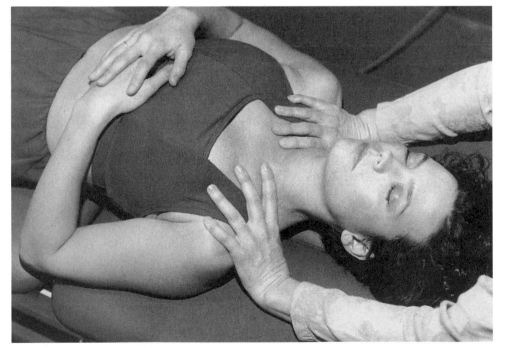

Figure 14-6: Thoracic inlet release.

The patient is supine. The therapist sits at the head of the table. Use a bilateral handhold on the clavicles, with thumbs on the superior aspect of the scapula as able. Motion test for anterior-posterior, superior-inferior, and rotational preference. Follow any strain patterns present in all three planes. You can access the entire thorax through this hold and release. The thoracic inlet is important to evaluate with circulatory and lymphatic drainage dysfunction.

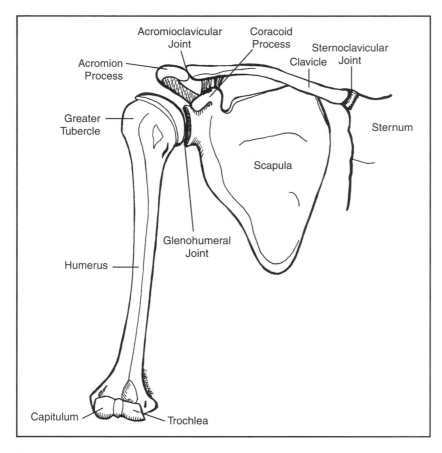

Figure 14-7A: Shoulder joint (anterior view).

Figure 14-7A shows an anterior view of the shoulder joint with ligaments at the sternoclavicular (S/C) and acromioclavicular (A/C) joints. Figure 14-7B is a posterior view of the shoulder. These drawings provide an anatomical reference for releases shown in Figures 14-8 and 14-9.

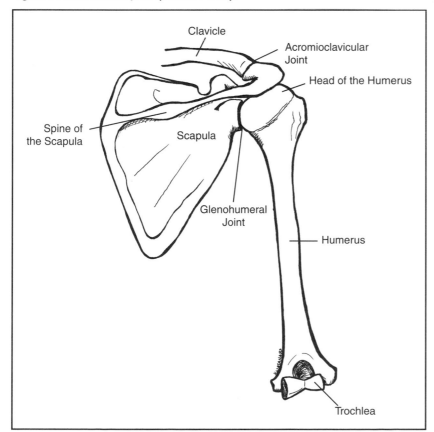

Figure 14-7B: Shoulder joint (posterior view).

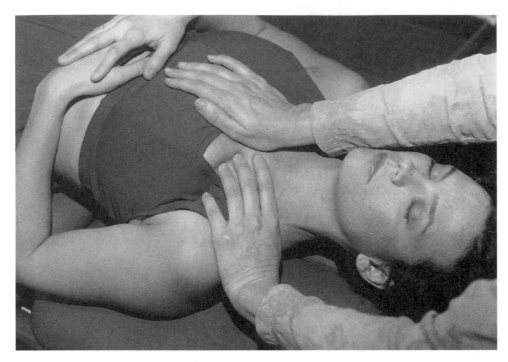

The patient is supine. The therapist sits at the head of the table. One hand stabilizes the sternum as the other hand mobilizes the clavicle. Motion test for anterior-posterior, superior-inferior, and rotational preference. Take the patient into motion of ease by broad surface contact along the clavicle. Again, motions can be stacked or done individually.

Figure 14-8: Sternoclavicular joint release.

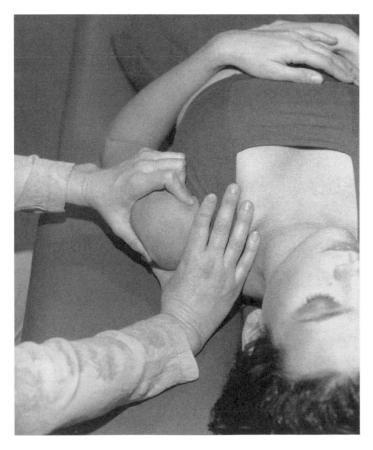

The patient is supine. The therapist sits or stands on the involved side, close to shoulder joint. Motion test for glenohumeral anterior-posterior, superior-inferior (compression distraction), and internal-external rotation preference. Stabilize proximally with one hand and take the humerus into the preferred motion with the other hand. Stack motions, if desired.

Figure 14-9: Glenohumeral joint release.

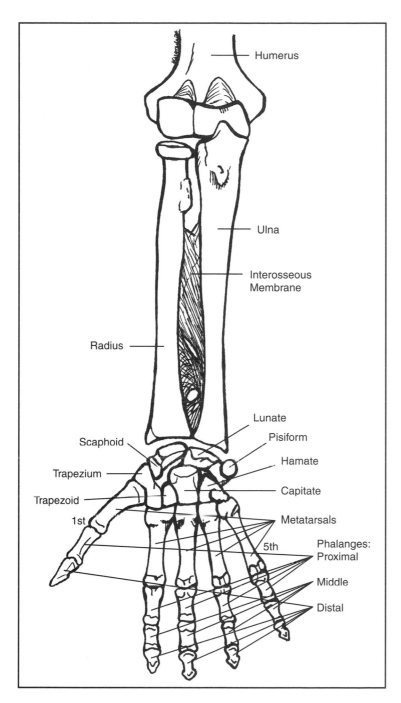

Figure 14-10: Elbow, wrist, and hand joints (anterior view).

Figure 14-10 shows an anterior view of the elbow, wrist, hand, and finger joints as well as the radius, ulna, and interosseous membrane. This drawing provides an anatomical reference for releases show in Figures 14-11 through 14-16.

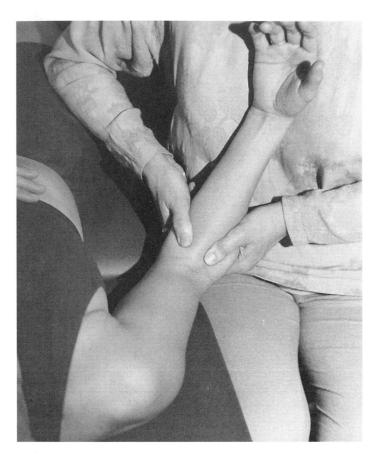

Figure 14-11: Superior radial-ulnar release.

The patient is supine. The therapist sits on the involved side. One hand stabilizes the ulna as the other hand mobilizes the radial head in an anterior-posterior direction. Fine tune the release using the rotational component (supination-pronation) and longitudinal compression or distraction through the radius, as needed, to release.

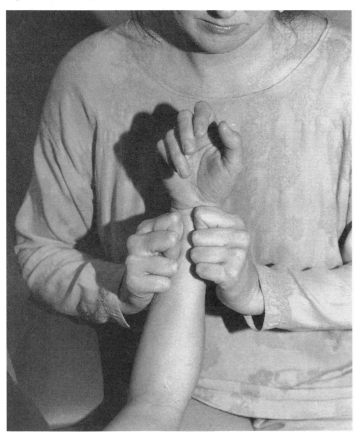

Figure 14-12: Inferior radial-ulnar release.

The patient is supine. The therapist sits on the involved side. One hand stabilizes the radius as the other hand mobilizes the ulna in an anterior-posterior direction. Fine tune the release using the rotational, compression, or distraction components. Take the patient into the preferred position and hold for the release.

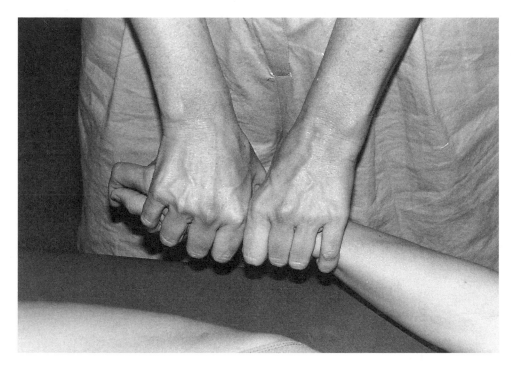

The patient is supine. The therapist stands on the same side with elbows straight. Stabilize the radius with the web space of one hand as the other hand mobilizes the proximal row of carpal bones in an anterior-posterior direction. Take the patient into the preferred position to release. Fine tune the release with supination-pronation and radial-ulnar deviation.

Figure 14-13: Radial-carpal release.

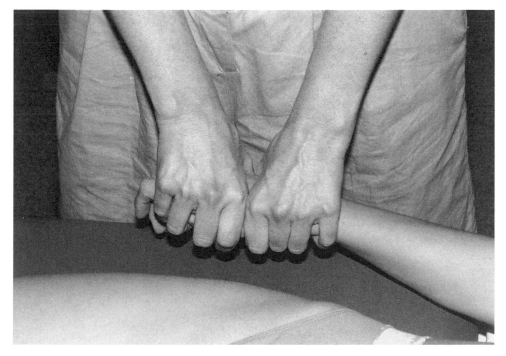

The patient is supine. The therapist stands on the same side with elbows straight. This release is similar to the radial-carpal release. Stabilize the proximal row of carpal bones with one hand while the other hand mobilizes the distal row of carpal bones. Assess for anterior-posterior motion and release in the preferred position. Use rotational, compression, or distraction components to fine tune the release.

Figure 14-14: Mid-carpal joints release.

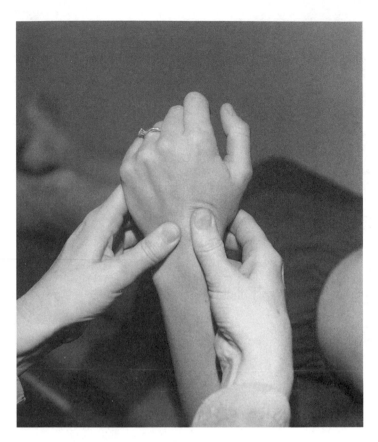

The patient is supine. The therapist sits on the involved side. Stabilize one carpal bone, such as capitate (shown). Mobilize the adjacent articulations, such as the trapezoid, scaphoid, lunate, and hamate bones. Assess the anterior-posterior motion and release by exaggerating the preferred position. Add any rotation, compression, or distraction components needed to fine tune the release. Use a flexion, extension, or other bias before doing the release, if necessary. Many variations of this release are possible for all carpal bone articulations.

Figure 14-15: Intercarpal joints release.

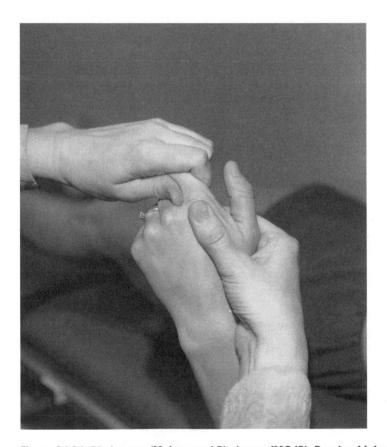

The patient is supine or sitting. The therapist sits on the involved side. One hand stabilizes the metacarpal bone and the other hand mobilizes the corresponding proximal phalange joint. Motion test for anterior-posterior, abduction-adduction, and rotational preference. Add compression or distraction, as necessary, to release in the preferred position.

Figure 14-16: Phalanges (Metacarpal Phalange (MC/P), Proximal Interphalange (PIP), and Distal Interphalange (DIP)) release.

Reference

1. Kain K with Berns J. *Ortho-Bionomy®: A Practical Manual.* Berkeley, CA: North Atlantic Books; 1997.

15

Lumbar and Thoracic Spine Joint Application

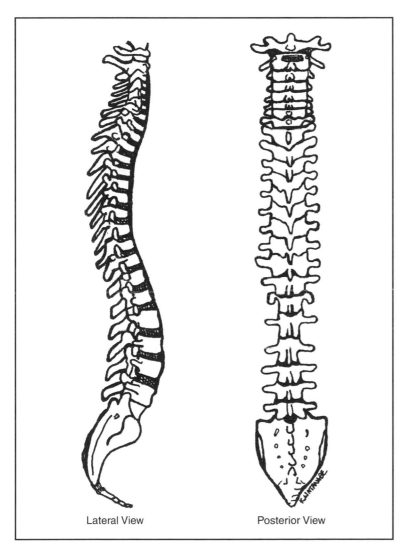

Figure 15-1A shows a lateral view of the thoracic and lumbar spine and Figure 15-1B shows a posterior view of the spine. These drawings provide a general anatomical reference for the releases shown in Figures 15-2 through 15-4.

Lateral View   Posterior View

Figure 15-1A: Spine (lateral and posterior views).

Prone, side-lying, and sitting releases are used for restrictions found in the lumbar or thoracic spine. Motion test to determine the segmental restrictions, using hip flexion or extension on the involved side. This is done most easily in the side-lying position with the involved side up or in a sitting, rather than prone, position.

First consider whether the segmental dysfunction is in a flexed or extended position and recreate the position of comfort and ease of motion with your release. From here, add the side-bending and rotation components. For learning purposes, these applications are separated into individual release positions, but best results will be obtained by stacking the releases.

The prone extension, rotation, and side-bending releases as well as flexion (leg off the table) releases are used primarily for lumbar spine dysfunctions. However, they also can be used for lower to mid-thoracic spine dysfunctions. Address mid- and upper thoracic spine dysfunctions with rib lift (Figure 15-2C) and side-bending releases using the arms overhead (Figure 15-2F), with the patient in a prone position. Side-lying releases are best used to address lumbar and lower thoracic spine dysfunctions.

Sitting releases address the entire lumbar and thoracic spine in a highly functional position. For upper thoracic spine (T_1–T_4) use the head only and passively flex, extend, side bend, or rotate to level. For a patient with a forward head posture, you may need to use a dorsal glide (chin tuck) to localize to the correct level. Patients typically present with extension of the middle and upper cervical spine and flexion of the lower cervical spine. If you attempt to use extension of the neck for the release, the movement will occur at the already extended (middle and upper) cervical segments. Likewise, if you attempt to use flexion of the neck for the release, the movement will occur in the lower cervical spine. Either way you will not be able to localize the upper thoracic spine segments you are attempting to address. A dorsal glide or chin tuck will lock out the cervical spine and movement will then occur in the thoracic region as intended.

For lower thoracic spine (T_5–T_{12}) and lumbar spine, the patient crosses one or both arms on the chest, as needed. The therapist uses one arm under or over the patient's crossed arm to motion test and position the patient, while the other hand palpates at the involved level. With sitting releases, start with patient in a straight or neutral spinal position. Try to maintain a central position by incorporating a translation into the release. Localize to the segmental level you are addressing by translating the spine from both above and below. Put the spinous process of the involved vertebrae perpendicular to the floor. Determine if the preferred position is in flexion or extension first, then add side-bending and rotation components by translation through the trunk and shoulders. The side-bending component is done most easily from opposite side as described later. Again, motions should be stacked to facilitate results.

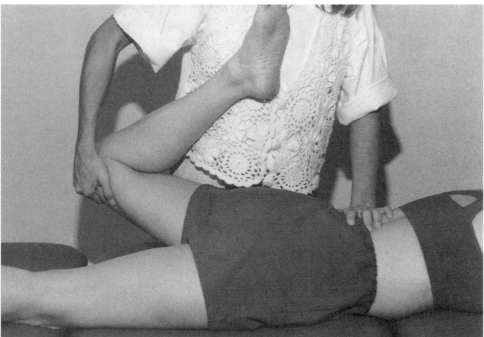

The patient is prone. The therapist stands on the involved side. One hand palpates the involved spinous or transverse process of the lumbar spine. The other hand lifts the hip into extension and adjusts the rotation and side-bending components, as needed. Position the hip in extension with pillows, if needed, then add ilium lift, single-leg rotation and side-bending aspects of the release.[1]

Figure 15-2A: Lumbar and thoracic prone extension release.

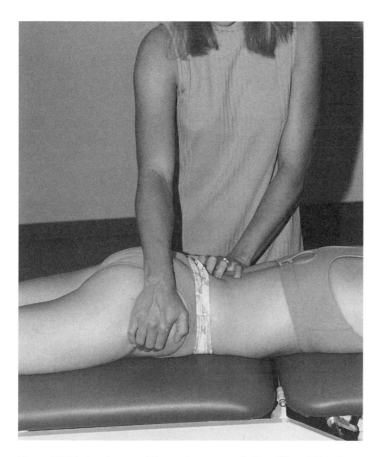

The patient is prone. The therapist stands on the side opposite to the involved side and lifts the hip to create the desired amount of spinal extension. One hand palpates the lumbar spine along the involved spinous or transverse process. The other hand lifts the ilium posterior and medial with pelvic rotation until you find a position of ease in lumbar spine.[1]

Figure 15-2B: Lumbar and thoracic prone rotation (ilium lift) release.

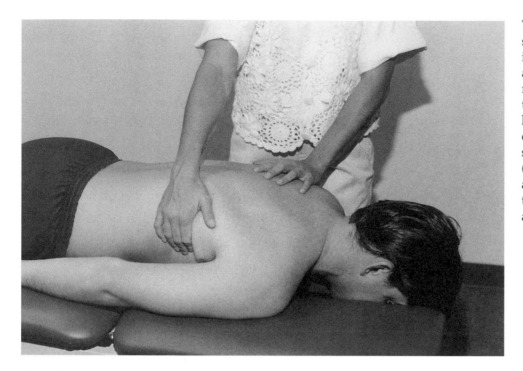

Figure 15-2C: Thoracic prone rotation (rib lift).

The patient is prone. The therapist stands on the side opposite to the involved side. To create the desired amount of thoracic spine extension, raise the head of the table or position the thorax on pillows. One hand palpates the involved spinous or transverse process of thoracic spine. The other hand lifts the ribs (or scapula) toward the involved area. If scoliosis is present, follow the curves to find ease of motion and a release position.[1]

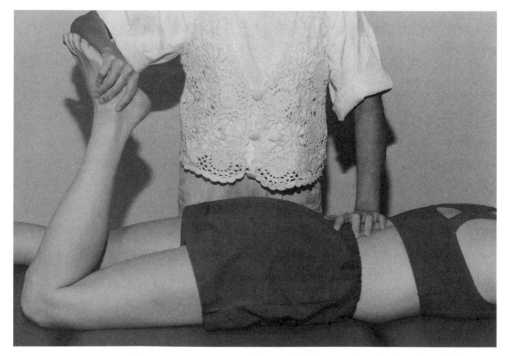

Figure 15-2D: Lumbar and thoracic prone single-leg rotation release.

The patient is prone. The therapist stands on the side opposite the involved side and extends the hip to create the desired amount of spinal extension. One hand palpates lumbar spine along the involved spinous or transverse processes. The other hand takes the leg into approximately 90° of knee flexion and rotates the hip, knee, and ankle into varying degrees of flexion and rotation to find the position of ease, which decreases point tenderness. Use ankle rotation to fine tune the release.[1]

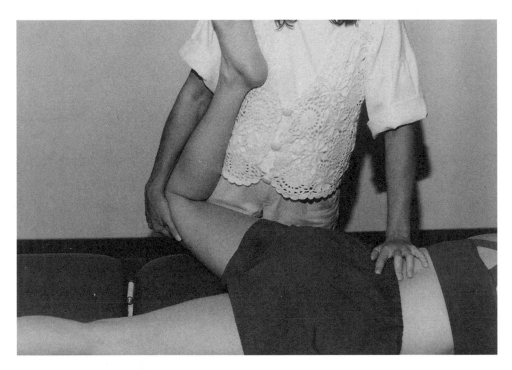

The patient is prone. The therapist stands on the involved side and extends the hip to create the desired amount of spinal extension. One hand palpates the involved spinous or transverse process of the lumbar spine. The other hand takes the hip into abduction to increase the side-bending component.

Figure 15-2E: Lumbar and thoracic prone side-bending release (using the leg).

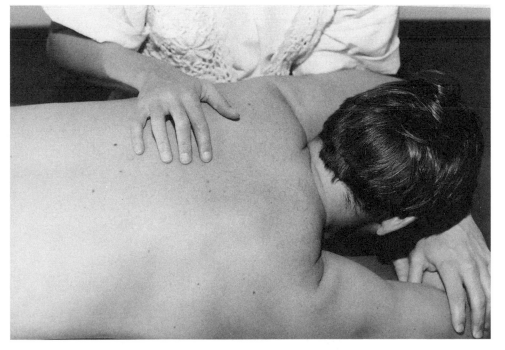

The patient is prone with arms straight and crossed overhead or the head resting on arms with elbows bent. The therapist stands on the involved side and places one arm under the patient's arms. Slide the patient toward you to increase the side-bending component. This release position, with arms overhead, will increase the extension in the thoracic spine. A more neutral spine position can be obtained by lowering the head of the table.

Figure 15-2F: Thoracic prone side-bending release (using the arms).

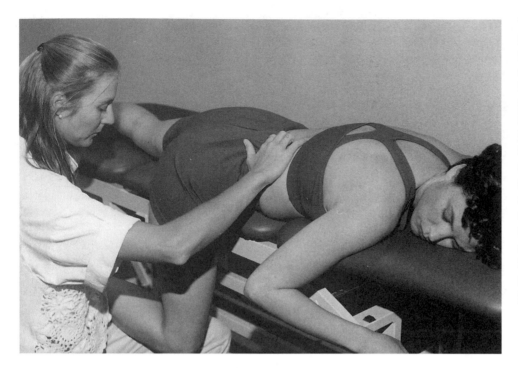

Figure 15-2G: Lumbar and thoracic prone flexion release.

The patient is prone with the involved-side leg lowered off the table. The therapist sits on a low stool on same side (or raises table). One hand palpates the involved spinous or transverse process of the lumbar spine. The other hand controls the leg off the table with varying degrees of flexion (hip and knee flexion), rotation (hip internal-external rotation), and side-bending (hip abduction-adduction). Fine tune the release through ankle motion. This release is useful if the original injury occurred while the spine was in a flexed position and anterior involvement (psoas, abdominals, etc.) is present.[1]

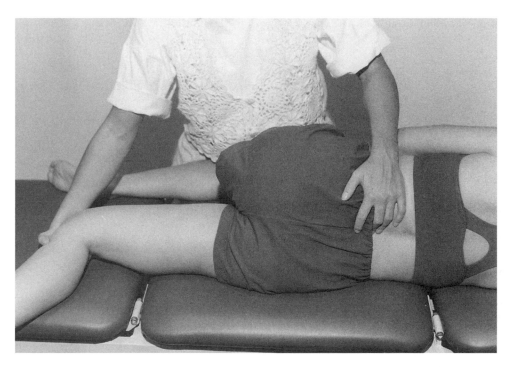

Figure 15-3A: Lumbar and lower thoracic side-lying extension release.

The patient is side-lying with legs straight and the involved side up. The therapist stands in front of the patient. Rest the upper leg in front of the lower leg. One hand palpates the involved spinous or transverse process of lumbar spine. The other hand passively extends the lower leg to the involved level for the release.

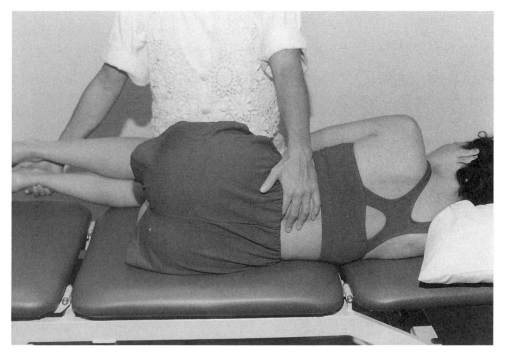

Figure 15-3B: Lumbar and lower thoracic side-lying flexion release.

The patient is side-lying with both legs flexed and the involved side up. The therapist stands in front of the patient. One hand palpates the involved spinous or transverse process of the lumbar spine. Both knees rest in the pelvic pocket of therapist. Flex the legs to the involved level for the release.

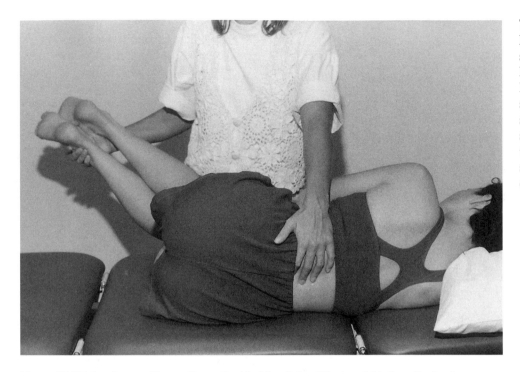

The patient is side-lying with 90° of hip and knee flexion. The therapist stands in front of the patient. Motion test by lifting both lower legs up toward ceiling to assess the side-bending component. Switch sides to test side-bending to opposite side. Flex or extend the legs to the level of involvement and add a side-bending component by raising or lowering both legs.

Figure 15-3C: Lumbar and lower thoracic side-lying lateral flexion (side-bending) release.

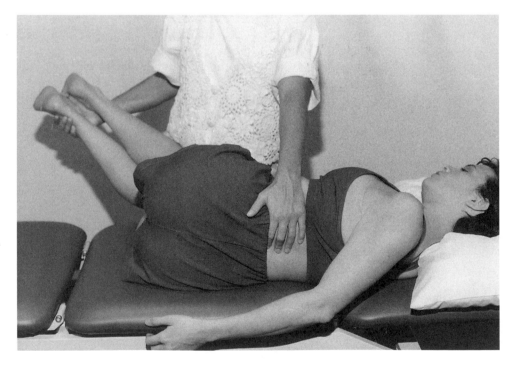

The patient is side-lying. The therapist stands in front of the patient. Add a rotational component to the previous releases by posterior rotation of the trunk with the anterior rotation of the pelvis (shown) or anterior rotation of the trunk with the posterior rotation of the pelvis, while palpating at the involved level.

Figure 15-3D: Lumbar and lower thoracic side-lying rotation release.

The patient is sitting with the feet supported and one or both arms crossed on the chest. The therapist stands or sits close to the patient with one hand used to palpate the level of vertebral involvement and the other hand controlling the patient's trunk motion. Have the patient slowly slump or flex the spine to the level of involvement.

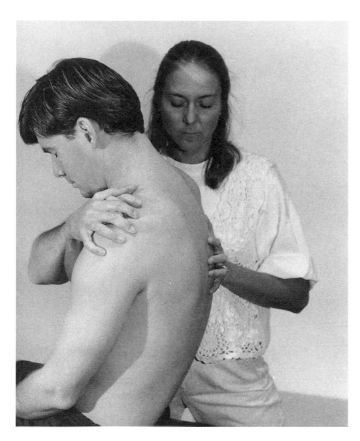

Figure 15-4A: Sitting flexion of lower thoracic and lumbar spine release.

The patient sits with the feet supported and one or both arms crossed over the chest. The therapist stands or sits with the palpating and moving hands as for the flexion release. Instruct the patient to assist by moving his or her umbilicus forward to increase the extension component. Extend the spine to the level of involvement.

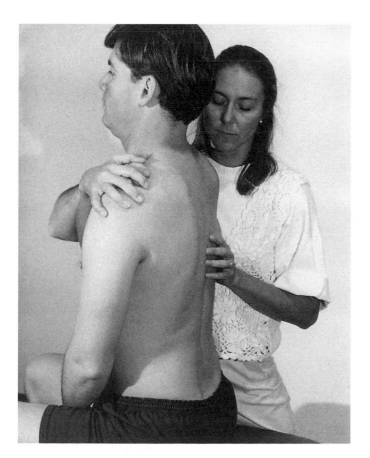

Figure 15-4B: Sitting extension of lower thoracic and lumbar spine release.

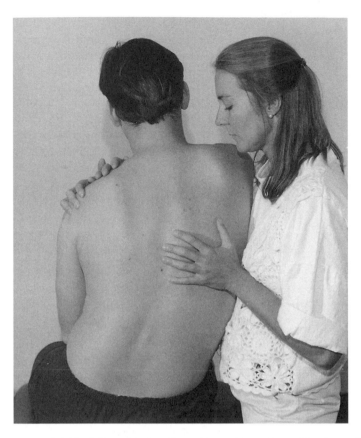

Figure 15-4C: Sitting side-bending of lower thoracic and lumbar spine release.

The patient is sitting with the feet supported and the arms crossed, as before. The therapist needs to stand or sit opposite the side to which you plan to side-bend toward to facilitate ease of patient handling. It is much easier to translate the patient toward you by inferior pressure on the opposite shoulder, as shown. Motion test left and right side-bending to determine the ease of motion preference prior to doing the release.

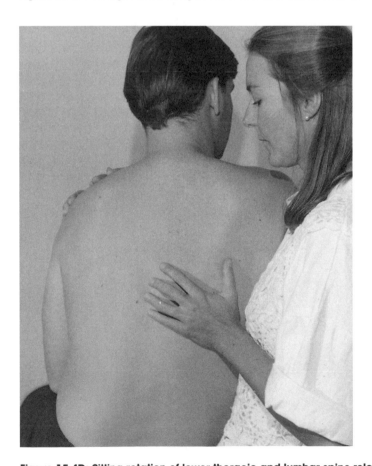

Figure 15-4D: Sitting rotation of lower thoracic and lumbar spine release.

The patient is sitting with the feet supported and arms crossed, as before. The therapist stands or sits on either side. Rotational motion is easier to do toward or away as compared to the side-bending motion. Patient handling is improved by close contact with the patient and control of the rotational motion through the opposite shoulder, as shown.

The patient is sitting with the feet supported on the floor or a stool. The therapist stands on the involved side. Flex the neck to the level of involvement and add side-bending and rotation to the same or opposite side to release. Use a dorsal glide (chin tuck) prior to release if necessary to lock out cervical spine motion. Releases shown in Figures 15-4E–H can also be used to address cervical spine dysfunction.

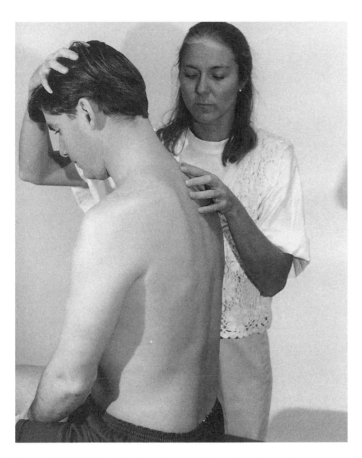

Figure 15-4E: Sitting flexion of upper thoracic spine release.

The patient is sitting with the feet supported on the floor or a stool. The therapist stands on the involved side. Extend the neck to the level of involvement with chin tuck, as needed, to lock out cervical spine motion. Add side-bending and rotation components to the same or opposite side as you palpate for the release position.

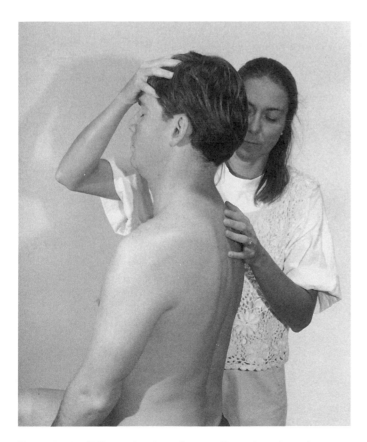

Figure 15-4F: Sitting extension of upper thoracic spine release.

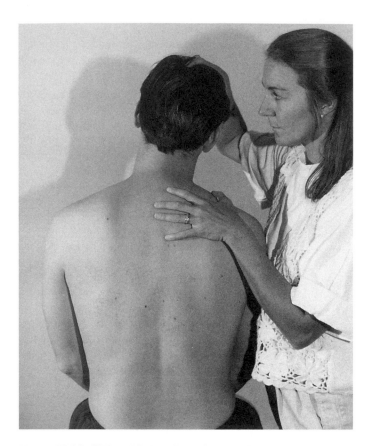

The patient is sitting. The therapist stands on the involved side and flexes or extends the neck to the level of involvement. Laterally flex the neck toward or away from the involved side as you palpate for the release position.

Figure 15-4G: Sitting side-bending of upper thoracic spine release.

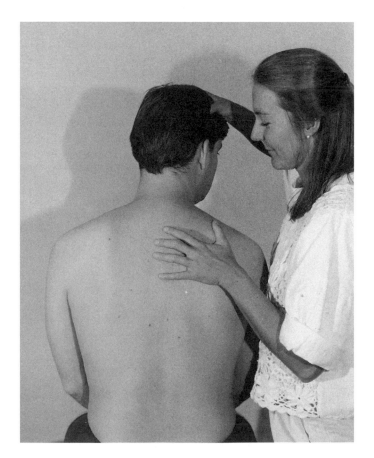

Patient is sitting. Therapist stands on involved side and flexes or extends to level of involvement. Rotate neck towards or away from involved side as you palpate for the release position.

Figure 15-4H: Sitting rotation of upper thoracic spine release.

Reference

1. Kain K with Berns J. *Ortho-Bionomy®: A Practical Manual.* Berkeley, CA: North Atlantic Books; 1997.

16

Cervical Spine Joint Application

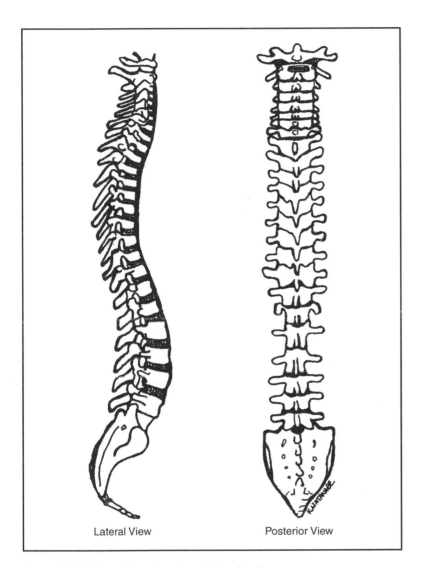

Figure 16-1 (left) shows a lateral view of the spine and Figure 16-1 (right) shows a posterior view. These drawings provide a general anatomical reference for Figures 16-2 through 16-7.

Lateral View

Posterior View

Figure 16-1: Spine (lateral and posterior views).

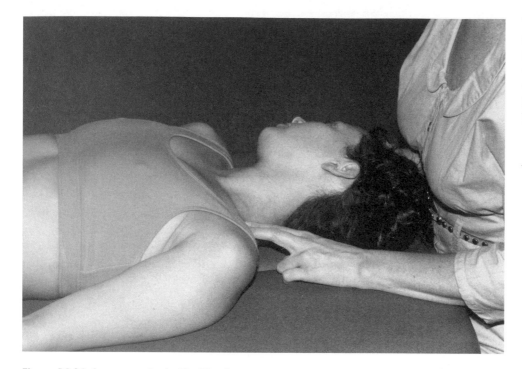

Figure 16-2A: Lower cervicals (C$_6$-T$_1$) release.

The patient is supine. The therapist sits at the head of the table. Palpate for triggers anterior to the transverse processes of lower cervicals with one hand, while the other hand rotates head away from side being released (Figure 16-2A).

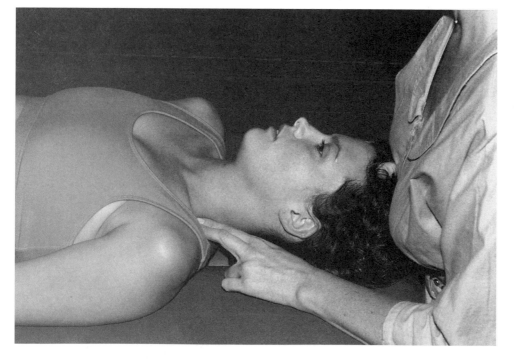

Figure 16-2B: Lower cervicals (C$_6$-T$_1$) release.

Laterally glide the neck toward the trigger to isolate the vertebrae you are releasing. Derotate the neck back towards the release point slowly (Figure 16-2B). The release position usually will be found before reaching the midline.[1]

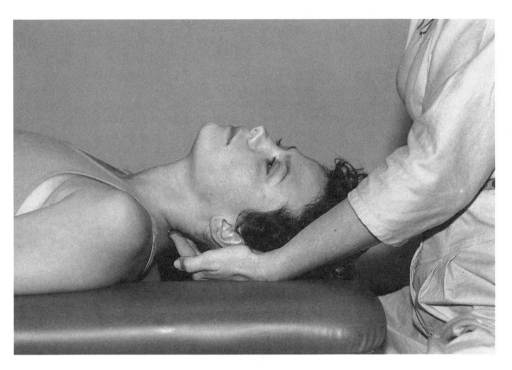

Figure 16-3: Mid-cervicals (C₂-C₆) extension release.

The patient is supine. The therapist sits at the head of the table. Use this release for periosteal or myofascial trigger points located on or around the spinous process or posterior to the transverse processes. One hand palpates the trigger as the other hand takes the neck into extension with side-bending and rotation, usually to the same side. If this is not the position of ease, try any combination of rotation and side-bending that decreases point tenderness. Occasionally, you may need to take the head off the table to get enough extension to obtain the release. See the discussion of the upper trapezius release in Chapter 10 and Figure 10-3B for the head-off-the-table procedure.[1]

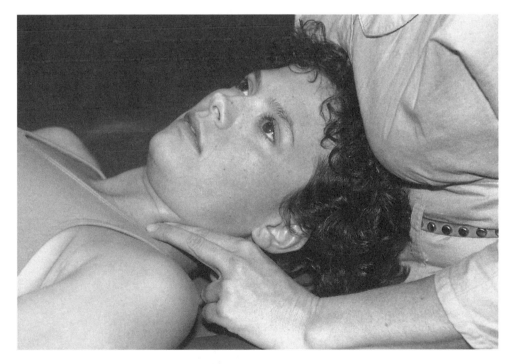

Figure 16-4: Mid-cervicals (C₂-C₆) flexion release.

The patient is supine. The therapist sits at the head of the table. Use this release for periosteal or myofascial trigger points located anterior to the transverse processes. One hand palpates the trigger as the other hand takes the neck into flexion with side-bending and rotation to the same or opposite side. Follow the patient's unique pattern for their ideal release position.

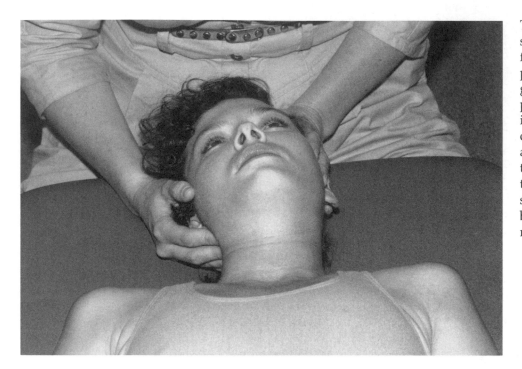

Figure 16-5: Occiput-atlas release.

The patient is supine. The therapist sits at the head of the table. Palpate for the trigger on the C_1 transverse process. Motion test C_1 for lateral glide. The involved side usually is point tender and lateral glide is limited toward opposite side. To release, one hand palpates the trigger on C_1 and the other hand laterally glides the C_1 transverse process toward the trigger. With a lateral glide to one side, add slight rotation and side-bending to the opposite side for the release.[1]

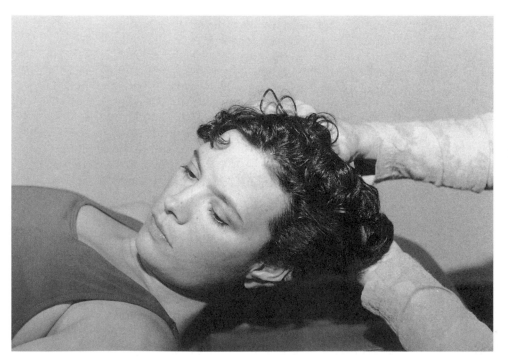

Figure 16-6: Atlas-axis (C_1–C_2) release.

The patient is supine. The therapist stands at the head of the table. Maximally flex the cervical spine (to 45° or more) to lock out the lower cervical spine. Assess the motion by right and left rotation and determine any restriction and the direction of ease. Take the patient into the preferred rotation and hold for the release.

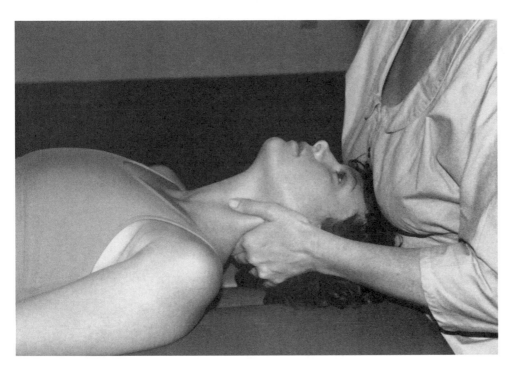

Figure 16-7A: Cervical spine extension release.

The patient is supine. The therapist sits at the head of the table. Find the area of greatest restriction by palpating differences at interspinous spaces and by motion testing using the transverse process handhold. Assess motion in all three planes with flexion and extension, side-bending right and left, and rotation right and left. Movement is away from the barrier and into the ease of motion. Isolate the involved segment by flexing or extending to the level, then add the side-bending and rotation components when stacking motions. Motions also can be done singularly in one plane of motion, as shown in Figures 16-7A–D.

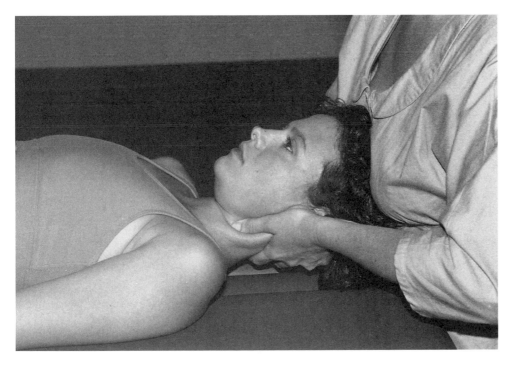

Figure 16-7B: Cervical spine flexion release.

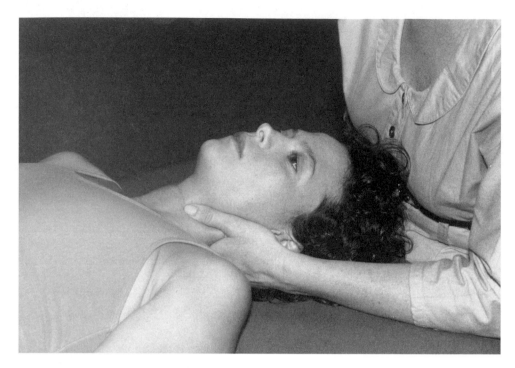

Figure 16-7C: Cervical spine side-bending release.

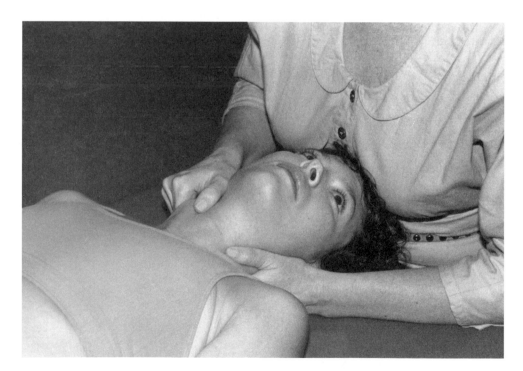

Figure 16-7D: Cervical spine rotation release.

Reference

1. Kain K with Berns J. *Ortho-Bionomy®: A Practical Manual.* Berkeley, CA: North Atlantic Books, 1997.

17

Isometrics

Theoretical Basis

Korr is credited with the theoretical basis for the isometrics presented in this Positional Release book.[1] He discussed the use of isometrics with both hypertonic muscles, as with muscle energy techniques, and their antagonist, as with Positional Release isometrics. In "Proprioceptors and Somatic Dysfunction," he stated,

> Apparently similar results may be obtained by eliciting isometric contractions, not of the hypertonic muscles, but of their antagonists. In this procedure, the physician is, of course, utilizing the principle of reciprocal innervation. The inhibitory influence of this mechanism, like that of the tendon receptors, may also be expected to affect the gamma as well as the alpha motoneurons.[1]

This is compared to the use of isometrics that relies on the principle of maximum relaxation following maximum contraction, as with muscle energy or proprioceptive neuromuscular facilitation (PNF) contract-relax techniques.[2]

Several additional benefits are thought to occur with the use of isometrics with Positional Release techniques. Isometrics are thought to improve the balance of tone between the agonist and antagoist muscles by increasing the tone in the hypotonic or overstretched muscle and promoting relaxation of the hypertonic or shortened muscle. This improved muscle balance and optimal tone should help increase the stability of the associated joints. Isometrics also are thought to begin the muscle reeducation process, through recruitment and activation of less active muscle fibers. Following the release and isometric with gentle oscillatory or other movements in the newly available range of motion will further the neuromuscular reeducation process, as the muscles are able to experience and remember (perhaps, forgotten) movement possibilities.

For comparative purposes, isometric exercises are not part of Strain-CounterStrain® or Functional technique procedures.[3,4] Osteopathic reference to isometrics usually focuses on muscle energy techniques, which involve a different theoretical basis, as mentioned previously. Isometrics and isotonic exercises are part of Ortho-Bionomy® practice.[5]

Isometric Procedure

At times, doing an isometric following each single release is the appropriate intervention. An alternative method of working is to do several releases in the target area, and after a certain amount of resolution of soft tissue or joint dysfunction has occurred, follow up with several isometrics. In any case, the point is to begin with the release process and end with isometrics and gentle movements to further the neuromuscular reeducation process, as mentioned. The release process is not reviewed here but refer to Chapter 7 for muscular releases and Chapter 12 for joint releases.

Begin the isometric from the release position or modify to a more neutral position if necessary. This will engage the antagonist to the released muscle groups. If you intend to follow a given release with an isometric, think about your hand position, body mechanics, and ability to provide resistance to their muscular contraction. You may need to modify your contact slightly but generally should be in the correct position for isometrics following the release. Ask the patient to contract the target antagonist, giving verbal and tactile cues. Stay specific to recruit the desired fibers and avoid overflow to other areas. The ideal isometric exercise is a submaximal contraction of specific target motor units. The isometric should be held for 6–10 counts, after the exact recruitment of fibers has been obtained.

It is important to follow the isometric contraction with a few gentle oscillatory-type movements to integrate the newly available range of motion into the client's awareness. After the isometric, reassess the target muscle point tenderness or joint range of motion through mobilization. Repeat the release and the isometric sequence, or only the isometric, as needed, with modification of the release and isometric based on the new assessment.

Isometric Applications

Isometrics can be very general or quite specific, based on the therapist's treatment goals, time constraints, and patient response. Doing a few general isometrics (shown at the end of this chapter) following releases of key areas, such as the pelvis, trunk, and target extremity or spinal area, often is beneficial in a short treatment time of 10–15 minutes. If you suspect a direct or relational involvement in a certain area other than your target area, a few general releases and isometrics are an excellent way to address the dysfunction without a large investment of time.

At the other end of the spectrum, it is possible to use isometrics in very specific ways to recruit target motor units in an area. This more specific work requires a little more time, patience, and skill but can be developed easily with practice. The specific use of isometrics can address even long-held spinal and other dysfunctions, by changing the firing and recruitment patterns in an area, which begins the functional reorganization process. Exact verbal and tactile cues are used to isolate and engage the motor units you wish to recruit. This may require several attempts to get the desired results.

Remember that, while only a few general isometrics are shown in this chapter, all releases previously presented can be followed with an isometric. When doing either a muscular or joint release, the release position then becomes the starting point for the isometric. An exception to this is if the release position is thought to be too extreme for the patient to tolerate a contraction or if the isometric contraction causes increased pain. In this case, simply reposition the body part closer to a neutral or midline position before asking the patient to do the isometric contraction.

Use of breathing as the isometric contraction is recommended for several muscular and joint releases in the thorax. This would be appropriate for the abdominal muscles, pectorals, scalenes, any rib or thoracic spine releases as well as all diaphragm releases. After the release, instructions would be given to take in a deep breath, as the patient comes out of the release position. Appropriate resistance is provided by the therapist, to obtain the desired isometric contraction of the diaphragm muscle.

At times, it may be appropriate to use visualization or instructions to engage eye movements with (or as) the isometrics. These methods can be used to increase the power of a weak isometric contraction with a patient who has difficulty recruiting muscle fibers. Similar cues may be given to decrease excessive overflow to other muscles and obtain a submaximal contraction with a patient who is engaging excessive muscular force in response to a request for an isometric. The visualization process also is helpful if attempting to recruit muscular response at a certain joint in the kinetic chain. For example, when having the patient do an isometric for internal or external rotation of the leg, have that patient see or feel the movement coming from the hip, knee, and or ankle. A verbal cue alone will engage firing in the area mentioned.

Summary

1. Assess the target area.
2. Perform the muscular, joint, or general release.
3. Do an isometric out of the release position.
4. Perform gentle integrative movements in the new range of motion.
5. Reassess the muscle point tenderness or joint range of motion.
6. Modify the release and isometric sequence and repeat as needed.

Isometrics

Refer to the previous sections on procedure and application for more specifics for all isometrics and follow the steps outlined in the above summary. Figures 17-1 through 17-19 provide examples of isometrics frequently used with Positional Release techniques.

Ankle dorsiflexion and eversion isometric is shown. Isometric for ankle plantarflexion or inversion can also be done (not shown).

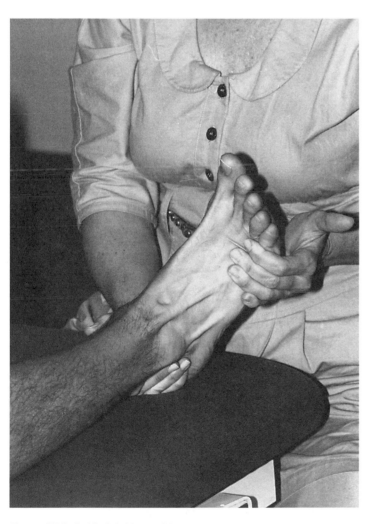

Figure 17-1: Ankle joint isometrics.

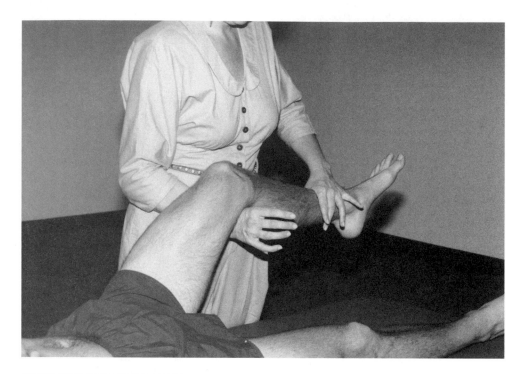

Knee extension isometric is shown. Knee flexion isometric can also be done (not shown).

Figure 17-2: Knee joint isometrics.

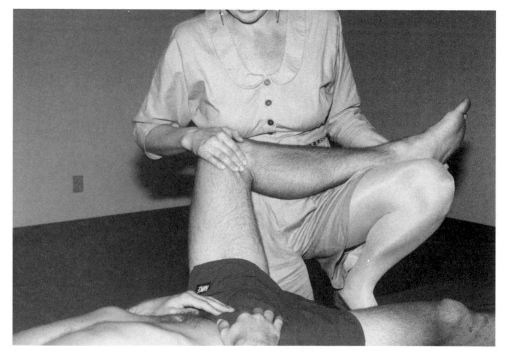

Hip internal rotation isometric is shown. Isometrics for hip external rotation, flexion, extension, abduction, or adduction can also be done (not shown).

Figure 17-3: Hip joint isometrics.

Right posterior and left anterior ilium rotation isometric is shown. This would follow release of right anterior or left posterior ilium.

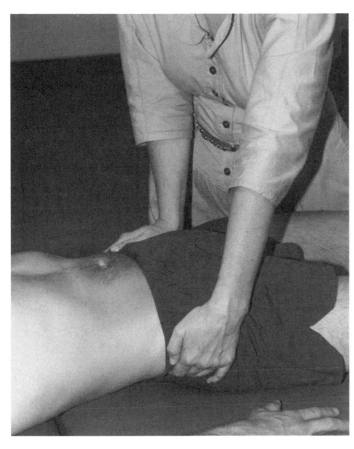

Figure 17-4: Pelvic isometric.

Left lateral rib and right lateral pelvic isometric is shown. This release and isometric are used for right lateral shift dysfunctions.

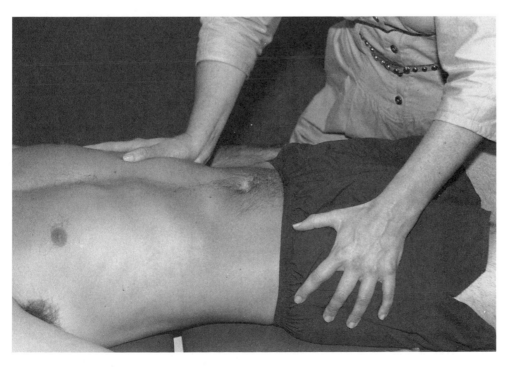

Figure 17-5: Rib-pelvis isometric.

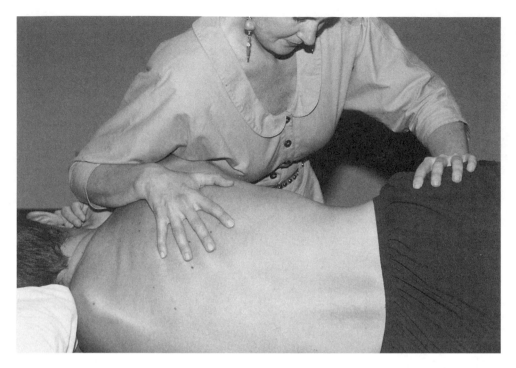

Posterior rotation of the trunk and anterior rotation of the pelvis isometric is shown. This would follow a release for an anterior trunk or posterior pelvic rotation.

Figure 17-6: Side-lying trunk-pelvis isometric.

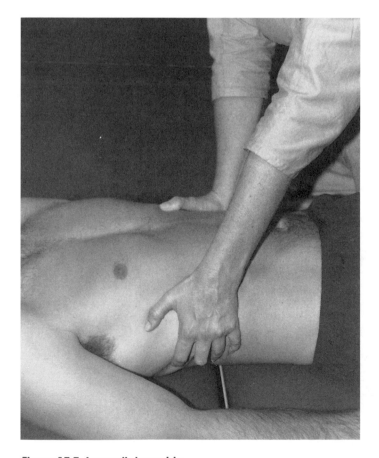

Right posterior and left anterior lower rib rotation isometric is shown. This would follow a release for a right anterior or left posterior rotation of the lower ribs.

Figure 17-7: Lower rib isometric.

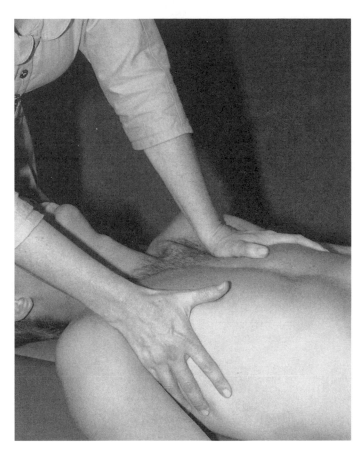

Figure 17-8: Upper rib isometric.

Left anterior and right posterior upper rib rotation isometric is shown. This would follow a release for right anterior or left posterior rib rotation.

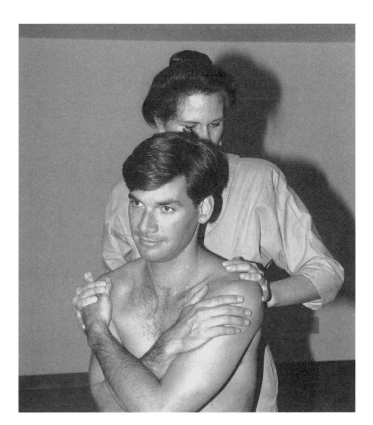

Figure 17-9: Sitting trunk rotation isometric.

Right anterior and left posterior trunk rotation isometric is shown in a sitting position. This would follow a release for left posterior or right anterior trunk rotation.

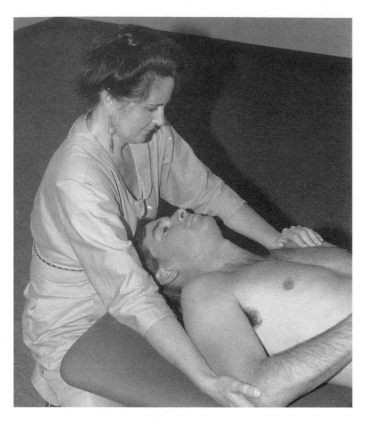

Figure 17-10: Superior-inferior shoulder girdle isometric.

Right inferior and left superior shoulder girdle isometric is shown. This would follow a release for right superior or left inferior shoulder girdle dysfunction.

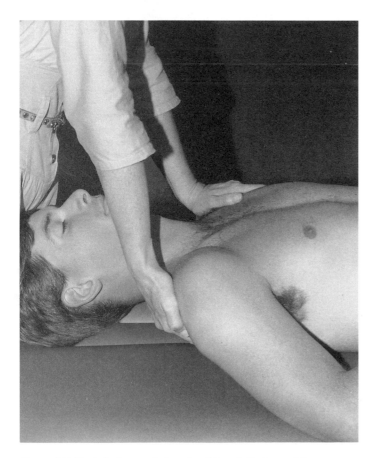

Figure 17-11: Anterior-posterior shoulder girdle isometric.

Right posterior and left anterior shoulder isometric is shown. This would follow a release for right anterior or left posterior shoulder girdle dysfunction.

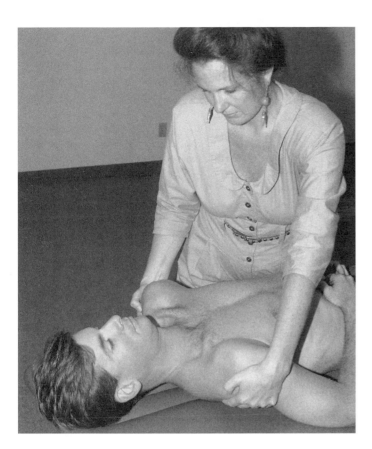

Figure 17-12: Bilateral forward shoulder isometric.

Bilateral posterior shoulder isometric (scapular retraction) is shown. This would follow a release for forward shoulders or scapular protraction.

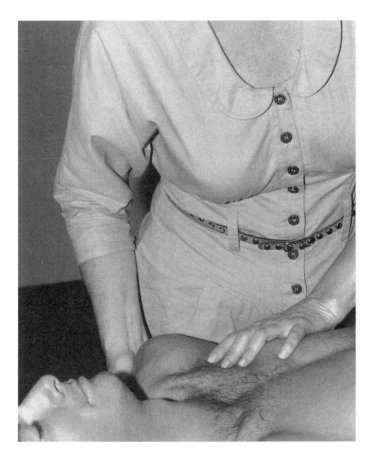

Figure 17-13: Shoulder joint isometrics.

Posterior shoulder joint isometric for anterior displacement is shown. Isometrics for shoulder internal or external rotation or posterior, superior, or inferior displacement can also be done (not shown).

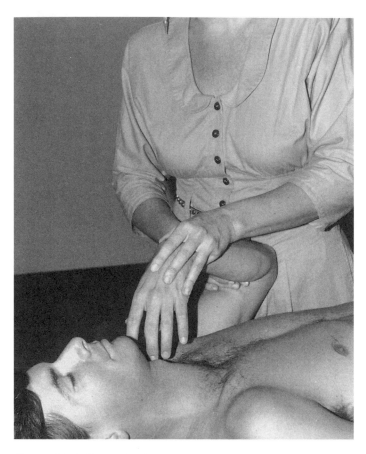

Figure 17-14: Elbow joint isometrics.

Elbow extension isometric is shown. Elbow flexion isometric can also be done (not shown).

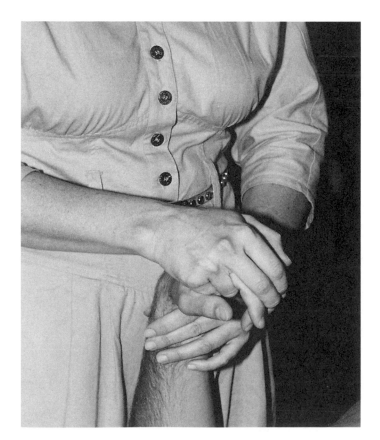

Figure 17-15: Wrist joint isometrics.

Wrist extension isometric is shown. Isometrics for wrist flexion, radial, or ulnar deviation can also be done (not shown).

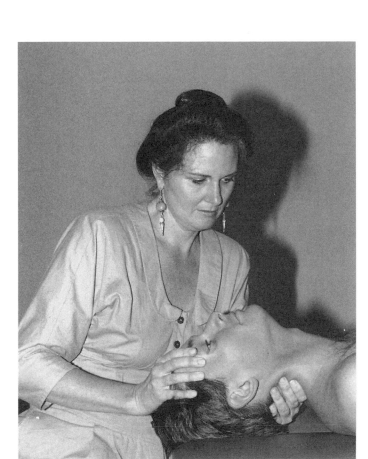

Neck flexion isometric following a release for neck extension is shown.

Figure 17-16: Cervical spine flexion isometric.

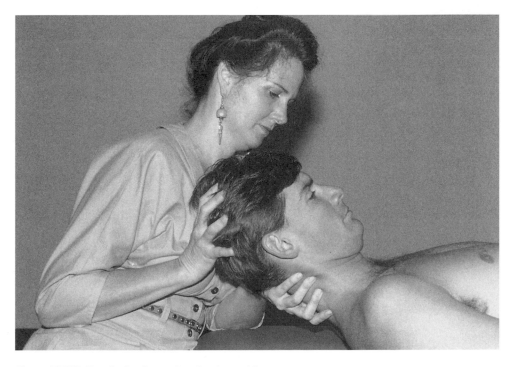

Neck extension isometric following a release for neck flexion is shown.

Figure 17-17: Cervical spine extension isometric.

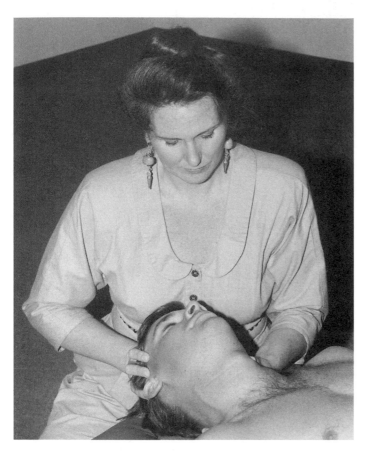

Figure 17-18: Cervical spine side-bending isometric.

Right lateral flexion or side-bending isometric following a release for left side-bending is shown.

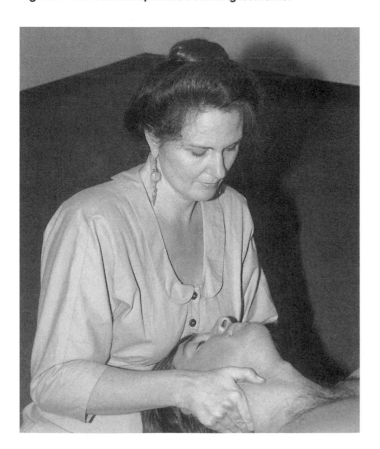

Figure 17-19: Cervical spine rotation isometric.

Right neck rotation isometric following a release for left rotation is shown.

References

1. Korr IM. Proprioceptors and somatic dysfunction. *Osteopathic Annals.* August 1974.
2. Knott M, Voss DE. *Proprioceptive Neuromuscular Facilitation.* 2nd ed. New York: Harper & Row; 1968.
3. Jones LH, with Kusunose RS, Goering EK. *Jones Strain-CounterStrain®.* Boise, ID: Jones Strain-CounterStrain; 1995.
4. Johnston WL, Friedman HD. *Functional Methods: A Manual for Palpatory Skill Development in Osteopathic Examination and Manipulation of Motor Function.* Indianapolis: American Academy of Osteopathy; 1994.
5. Kain K with Berns J. *Ortho-Bionomy®: A Practical Manual.* Berkeley, CA: North Atlantic Books; 1997.

Part III

Clinical Case Studies

Seven of the following case studies were done by University of Indianapolis postprofessional students enrolled in PT 535, Positional Release Techniques course, which fulfilled part of their requirements towards a Masters of Health Science or Masters of Science Degree in Physical Therapy. Requirements for this course included a three-day lab practicum in Positional Release and a postcourse case study in which Positional Release was used as part of the patient's treatment protocol. Case studies were edited by the author for format consistency and grammar, without any intentional change of content. Therapists who wrote the case studies reviewed the edited version prior to publication. These students may or may not have had any previous experience with indirect techniques or manual therapy. The final case study in Chapter 25 was done by the author. These case studies may provide some insight into the broad clinical application of Positional Release, integration with and comparison to other physical therapy techniques and potential outcome possibilities.

18

Case Study 1. Traumatic Cervical Spine Injury

Michelle Jones, P.T., MHS Program, University of Indianapolis
Edited comments by instructor Denise Deig, M.S.P.T., appear within rules.

Patient History and Subjective Information

The patient is a 30-year-old woman who presents severe posterior neck pain. The mechanism of injury was a hit by a softball to the posterior C_4–C_5 region during a coed softball game 12 hours prior to treatment. She was running toward home plate when she was struck in the back of the neck with the ball. The patient maintains a splinted neutral neck and shoulder posture throughout the treatment. She reports that neck movement in all directions is painful from 4–9/10 (with 10 being most severe).

The patient has been applying ice packs regularly and taking Advil every six hours. She kept a towel roll around her neck as a support that day at work while she typed and answered the phone. No other significant medical or traumatic history is reported.

Objective Findings

1. Cervical spine range of motion (ROM) is limited and painful in all directions.
2. Shoulder ROM is within normal limits bilaterally.
3. Scapular ROM is within normal limits (WNLs) bilaterally, but painful.
4. Manual muscle testing of neck, scapulae, and bilateral upper extremities is WNLs, with neck and upper back pain with neck, shoulder, and scapular motion.
5. Redness and edema noted over C_4 and C_5 region, with no bruising.
6. Posterior point tenderness noted bilaterally in upper trapezius, rhomboids, and levator scapulae on the left more than the right side.
7. Neurological exam found no abnormalities.

Treatment Goals

1. Increase ROM in cervical spine.
2. Decrease pain.
3. Improve awareness and patient education.
4. Increase strength using isometrics, as tolerated.

Treatment and Patient Response

Treatment 1

Evaluation is carried out. Positional Release is given to bilateral rhomboids, upper and middle trapezius, levator scapulae, and suboccipitals. Rhomboid and right upper trapezius point tenderness are 100% resolved. Left upper trapezius is improved by 25%. Neck rotation and lateral flexion are improved by 75%, flexion improved by 50%, and extension by 25%. Bilateral scapular ROM and pain are improved by 75%. The patient is told to continue with ice, Advil, and neck support and to limit extreme neck ROM as able. She is informed that pain and stiffness may return.

Treatment 2 (Day 2)

The patient reports that neck is tired and stiff but not as painful. She continues using Advil and needed ice only last evening. She did not use ice or neck support at work. Pain with motion is 2–5/10 except for neck extension, which is 6–7/10. The neck ROM is limited by 50% except for extension, which is limited by 75%. The posterior neck edema decreased by 25% with no bruising or redness noted. The posterior trigger points in the upper trapezius, rhomboids, and levator scapulae decreased in number and intensity by 50% on the left side and increased on the right. The treatment includes Positional Release followed by isometrics to bilateral levator scapulae, rhomboids, and upper and lower trapezius. The trigger points resolved 100% except for one on left T_3–T_4 area. The ROM is WNLs with pain decreased to 1/10 for all motions except extension, which is 3–4/10. Recommendations are given as on the previous day. The patient is instructed in gentle stretching of neck, shoulders, and scapula within a pain-free ROM.

Treatment 3

The patient canceled her appointment scheduled two days later, due to no complaint of pain or limitation of motion in any direction. The area of direct hit still is painful to touch and pressure. The home program for stretching is reviewed by phone and continued use of ice and Advil recommended.

One-Week Posttreatment

The patient reports she still is doing well, with a 75% improvement in touch and pressure response to her posterior neck. She reports no bruising to date and no return of pain or stiffness. She continues with stretching for only a couple of days after the last treatment.

Discussion

I am very pleased with the overall results I obtained with this patient. Particularly, I am glad to have a technique I feel comfortable using so early in the acute phase of this type of injury. I probably would not have treated this patient so quickly (12 hours post injury), prior to learning Positional Release. If I had treated this patient, I would have done only very mild passive ROM and continued with ice and antiinflammatories. I certainly would not have expected to see the extent of pain relief and increased ROM so quickly.

I am not surprised that pain persisted over the cervical site where the injury occurred. Due to the soft tissue injury, the body must have time to heal. By relieving the protective spasm and resulting pain, I feel this injury was a perfect example of how well Positional Release fits into practice.

I am comfortable with this technique because it is so nontraumatic. The patient was extremely comfortable because I did nothing to increase her pain. I put her in only positions that were pain free. I feel that patient compliance and positive results relate to patient comfort during the treatment sessions. Once she realized that the treatment was not going to be painful, it was noticeable how much more she relaxed. Her relaxation made it easier for me to find and follow the positions of comfort.

The first session took longer than I would have liked, but subsequent sessions using Positional Release became more comfortable as my knowledge and patient handling increased. I was so pleased with the results I almost could not believe it. I since have treated several patients using Positional Release. Some have had results as positive and some not as significant; however, improvements have been noted with each patient. I am sure that, as I get more proficient with my abilities, I will see more positive results.

This case study is an excellent example of how beneficial Positional Release can be with acute posttraumatic injury. How often do physical therapists see a patient 12 hours post trauma? I rarely have had such an opportunity. The length of treatment required is directly proportional to the chronicity of the dysfunction and the time since the injury occurred. In this case, only two visits were required for nearly complete resolution of the restrictions. With a quick intervention, such as described, the patient's own healing mechanism is speeded significantly and chronic holding patterns do not result due to the initial protective spasm lasting past an acute phase.

It is very significant that this therapist had the wisdom to instruct the patient in limiting extreme and painful motions. This demonstrates her knowledge of the potential danger of reducing the protective spasm early with an effective Positional Release intervention. Early intervention may be appropriate only with patients who demonstrate a high level of responsibility toward self-care. Otherwise, there is a potential for reinjury.

19

Case Study 2. Thoracic Outlet Syndrome

Wendel Lamason, P.T., MHS program, University of Indianapolis
Edited comments by instructor Denise Deig, M.S.P.T., appear within rules.

Patient History

The patient is a 31-year-old woman who was involved in a motor vehicle accident (MVA) on May 9, when her car was rear-ended. She experienced onset of left cervical, shoulder, scapular, anterior chest wall, and upper extremity pain at the time of the accident. The patient began having progressive left upper extremity paresthesia the first two weeks following the MVA. She had been working two jobs before the MVA, but had to stop working after the accident.

A magnetic resonance imaging (MRI) of the cervical spine found no abnormalities. Further testing with an angiogram revealed "normal vessels from the subclavian to the fingertips," per the physician's notes. However, the physician did report color changes in the left hand and decreased capillary refill when the shoulder was elevated to 90°. No medications were prescribed initially. The physician felt the condition resulted from seat belt impact.

The patient's past medical history was significant for a motorcycle accident in 1990, at which time she sustained a left clavicular fracture and other soft tissue injuries.

Subjective Information

Initially, the patient complained of left cervical, anterior chest wall, and scapular pain, reported to be constant with intermittent sharpness. Constant left upper extremity paresthesia (described as numbness, tingling, throbbing, coldness, and heaviness) also is reported. She relates an inability to lift her left arm overhead due to severe pain and tightness in the left shoulder girdle. She also mentions being unable to get sleep well or lift several objects at home.

Objective Findings

The patient previously had been seen at another physical therapy clinic for two or three visits, after which time she requested transfer to another facility, due to discomfort with her treating therapist. Due to scheduling circumstances, she was treated by another physical therapist for one week starting on June 8. Lamason became the primary therapist on June 17.

The initial therapist reported "poor tolerance to palpation" and a poor prognosis for recovery with physical therapy. Initially, cervical spinal range of motion was grossly limited by 75%. Left shoulder active range of motion (AROM) was limited to 85° flexion. Guarding was reported during range of motion (ROM) testing throughout the neck and left upper quarter. During the first two treatments, the patient was instructed in cervical spine ROM and isometric exercises.

Evaluation on June 17 revealed limited ROM of the cervical spine, with 25° of right rotation and 23° of left rotation. The ROM of left shoulder flexion is unchanged, with

75° of shoulder abduction measured. Gentle right cervical spine side-bending or rotation increases the symptoms in the left upper extremity. The patient is observed to be an upper chest breather when in a supine position. Functionally, the patient is unable to lift her purse with her left arm and reports an inability to lift objects such as pots, pans, and laundry basket.

Palpation on June 17 reveals multiple trigger points throughout the left sternocleidomastoid (SCM), scalenes, upper trapezius, supraspinatous, rhomboid, pectoralis, and deltoid muscles with suboccipitals tight and tender bilaterally. Superficial touch of the left anterior triangle and scalenes reproduce a "hard sharp pain," tingling paresthesia, and coldness in left arm that results in a guarded patient reaction for 2–3 minutes. Edema is noted over the left anterior triangle region as well. Also, an elevated left first rib is noted.

Treatment Goals

1. Increase ROM of the cervical spine.
2. Increase ROM of the left shoulder.
3. Decrease point tenderness in involved muscles and trigger points.
4. Decrease paresthesia in the left upper extremity.
5. Improve the breathing pattern.
6. Enhance independence in a home program and self-care activities.
7. Resume the previous level of function.

Treatment and Patient Response

Treatment 1

Initial evaluation is carried out. The patient reports a decrease in symptoms with the use of ice and is instructed to continue using ice at home. Positional Release techniques include treatment for suboccipitals, upper trapezius, and first rib. The patient was instructed in self-release for the first rib. Grade I transverse mobilizations are given to the cervical spine.

Treatment 2 (12 days later, due to scheduling)

The patient reports good short-term benefits from the initial home program. Shoulder flexion has increased to 120°, however she continues to have extremely guarded movements. During this treatment, an 80–90% reduction in symptoms is reported after Positional Release techniques, as already noted, in addition to left scalene release, diaphragmatic breathing instruction, and Feldenkrais®1 awareness work performed. The patient began taking a cortisone pack four to five days prior to this treatment session without success to date.

Treatment 3 (10 days later)

The patient reports good results with the home program of Positional Release, diaphragmatic breathing, Feldenkrais awareness exercises, and ice. Upper extremity symptoms now are reported to be intermittent rather than constant. AROM of left shoulder now is within normal limits (WNLs) throughout. The cervical spine ROM is increased to 40° for left rotation and 55° for right rotation. Trigger points and point tenderness continue but decrease after Positional Release activities. The patient reports a progressive reduction in symptoms to date in therapy, especially after "such gentle techniques" as Positional Release. Gentle shoulder shrugs, upper body ergometer, cervical isometrics, and therapeutic exercise for scapular reeducation are initiated as tolerated during this treatment session. These exercises are added to the home exercise program.

Treatments 4–9 (over a two-week period)

Treatment continued to consist of the above techniques in addition to progressive therapeutic exercises (PREs) and direct massage techniques. On session 9 cervical spinal rotation ROM was 55° bilaterally. Trigger points and point tenderness had resolved except for scalenes and upper trapezius. She was generally symptom free in left upper extremity except for intermittent mild tingling. Patient reports independence in all activities of daily living (ADLs). Left upper extremity strength is grossly 4/5 throughout. She is exercising 20 minutes at 3 mph on the treadmill and on the upper body ergometer for 10 minutes.

Treatments 10 and 11

The patient is scheduled for discharge on session 10 but complains of waking up with a "crick" in her neck. Cervical spinal rotation ROM is limited to 25° bilaterally. On palpation, acute trigger points are noted over bilateral SCMs and left scaleni muscles. The patient complains of a frontal headache. After two treatments of Positional Release techniques to these specific areas, along with direct soft tissue techniques, the cervical spinal ROM returns to its previous measure. Patient also is able to resume exercise and functional levels achieved prior to the flare-up.

Treatment 12

The patient is scheduled for a reevaluation and determination of return-to-work status in the following week.

Discussion

Since this patient is extremely guarded with multiple trigger points and increased upper extremity symptoms with superficial palpation to specific areas, I determined that she is an ideal candidate for strong incorporation of Positional Release techniques. She also presents poor breathing patterns, which is of initial concern. The patient attributes much of the therapy's success to "this gentle stuff" and states, "You did not hurt me like the last therapist did!"

This therapist demonstrates a very good and appropriate treatment progression from gentle indirect techniques to more direct massage techniques, as tolerated. Likewise with the exercise program, he progresses her from Feldenkrais[1] awareness work and diaphragmatic breathing to PREs. This is in contrast to the first physical therapist, who treated this patient with techniques that apparently were too aggressive for her tolerance, and she therefore discontinued that care. I also am bothered by a therapist who gives only exercises following a traumatic injury and, when the patient fails to respond, decides she has a poor prognosis. If a therapist lacks the skill to adequately treat a patient, the patient should be sent to a therapist who does. As in this case, the patient appears to enjoy a full recovery from the injury with proper intervention and she most likely will be able to return to work in a full capacity.

Reference

1. Rywerant Y. *The Feldenkrais Method: Teaching by Handling.* New Canaan, CT: Keats Publishing; 1983.

20

Case Study 3. Adolescent Idopathic Scoliosis

Tricia Mahoney, P.T., MHS Program, University of Indianapolis
Edited comments by instructor Denise Deig, M.S.P.T., appear within rules.

Patient History and Subjective Information

The patient is a 14-year-old female with a primary diagnosis of mid-scapular and low back pain secondary to an idopathic scoliotic curve measuring 47° in the thoracic region (convex on right) and 43° in the lumbar region (convex on left). No injury is reported, although the patient is very active in a number of sports, including basketball, softball, and soccer. There is no family history of scoliosis nor other significant medical history related to the spinal curve. The curve was diagnosed approximately one year prior to her initial therapy session.

The patient presented approximately three months ago complaining of mid-thoracic and lumbar pain, for which she had been undergoing therapeutic treatment weekly, consisting of moist heat or ultrasound or both, followed by a stretching and strengthening program focusing on the back and abdominal musculature, with minimal resolution of the discomfort. In addition, she had been placed in a Risser cast (nearly immobilizing the thoracic and lumbar spine) for six days, which was not tolerated well. The patient states that the cast decreases her pain somewhat but is too cumbersome and uncomfortable. The physician, therefore, returned her to her previous physical therapy program, already described, and stated that, in three months, she would be reevaluated for surgical intervention, if therapy was not successful.

Objective Findings

The evaluation consists of a visual postural assessment (with pictures), goniometric joint range of motion (ROM) measurements, and manual muscle testing. Strength of the abdominal musculature is evaluated, as it is noted to support the spine extrinsically.[1] Leg length is measured to detect any significant differences that could be related to the presentation. Skin mobility was assessed standing and supine. Spinal and sacroiliac movements are assessed with the patient standing, per muscle energy recommendations by Loren Rex, D.O. Reflexes and superficial pain sensation is checked to rule out neurological abnormalities. Examination for point tenderness is also completed.

The evaluation demonstrates the following:

1. Decreased strength of back and abdominal musculature with middle trapezius being the weakest at 3+/5 and other muscles at 4/5.
2. Straight leg raise limited to 80° bilaterally.
3. ROM within normal limits except for hip extension, –5° to –7° bilaterally.
4. Pain with lumbar spine extension, right side-bending, and rotation, with pain levels 5–8/10 (with 10 being most severe).
5. Posterior point tenderness on right T_1–T_9, with most severe being at T_4–T_7. Anterior point tenderness of right iliopsoas. Point tenderness rated 4–5/5.
6. Decreased skin mobility noted along concavity of lumbar curve, bilateral trapezius, thoracic and lumbar paraspinals, quadratus lumborum, psoas groups, and anterior fascial planes of thorax.

Treatment Goals

1. Decrease tissue immobility and pain.
2. Prepare the muscles for a gradual strengthening program.
3. Increase hip extension ROM.
4. Establish a home exercise program to improve posture (sitting and standing).
5. Continue athletic lifestyle with no limitations and decreased pain in back.

Treatment

Treatment 1

The patient evaluation is carried out. Moist heat is given prior to releases. Positional Release is given to diaphragm, right iliopsoas, and middle and lower trapezius.

Treatment 2

The point tenderness is reassessed and located at the anterior T_6, T_8, and L_1 vertebrae on the right, T_1–T_6 on the left, and L_2 and L_3 bilaterally. Moist heat is followed by Positional Release to the diaphragm, right serratus anterior and bilateral latissimus dorsi, and rhomboids. Myofascial release (direct) is given to the rhomboids following indirect work. Isometrics follow each release, as per patient tolerance.

Treatment 3

Point tenderness is noted left T_2 and L_1 and right L_5. Moist heat is followed by releases to the iliopsoas, diaphragm, trapezius, latissimus dorsi, serratus anterior, and sitting thoracic spine. Patient continues previous program of stretching and strengthening.

Treatments 4–6

The treatment continues, with reassessment, moist heat, and Positional Release to the involved areas. Also, the patient's home program is monitored for progress.

Patient Response

The patient's first response to Positional Release is amusing. Following a diaphragm release, she inquires as to when I would begin the treatment. She did not "feel" anything and so equates this to mean that nothing has been done. The same response occurs initially when the release techniques are performed on the iliopsoas. However, she responds favorably to the release after it is repeated, stating that her discomfort at the tender point has decreased from 4+/5 to 2/5. The same effect is realized on the posterior tender points with varied success. The patient seems to respond favorably to some releases, with decreased discomfort reported, more than others (notably the upper trapezius). The therapist notes changes in tissue mobility that would have led her to believe the patient's discomfort level is decreased but it is not reported to be. However, these muscles are in constant use in her athletic activities.

The patient's response to treatment improves over time, as noted by a decreased reliance on antiinflammatory medications and decreased soreness reported. Back discomfort increases following a week of increased athletic activity. She states when she uses her right upper extremity excessively, her pain is localized more to the right side. These acute trigger points seem to respond to Positional Release techniques much better than chronic areas. Direct myofascial techniques are enjoyed by the patient and improve tissue mobility but do not decrease point tenderness as much as Positional Release techniques.

Hip extension is increased by 3–4° and abdominal and trapezius strength increases. Tension still can be palpated in the right iliopsoas; however, the patient reports a decrease in point tenderness with palpation. Following the release techniques, the patient reports that many of her exercises are easier to do and do not cause the discomfort previously felt. Posture improves, with patient reporting being more erect with less fatigue. Improved endurance in sitting is noted.

The patient and her mother are instructed in release techniques for a home program and self-care. Following one week of working on the techniques, both stated that they are "getting the hang of it" as they come to understand the explanations given them regarding anatomy and biomechanics. During the last session, the patient stated she is refraining from participating in any sports until she returns to school, as she has tired of the activity and wants to "relax and enjoy the rest of the summer."

Discussion

Patients with scoliosis frequently face a limited choice in treatment options. Often, they are given braces or prepared for surgery, depending on the severity of the curve. Many physicians quote the research available when saying physical therapy is ineffective in the treatment of this condition. The patient described failed use of a cast and was not interested in orthotic intervention. She remains a candidate for possible surgical intervention. Her pain limits her ability to function in normal athletic activities. Although the initial three weeks of treatment described may be an appropriate length of therapy, the treating therapist's professional opinion is that this patient will continue to improve with weekly therapy sessions.

The Positional Release techniques are thought to have assisted her in performing the exercise program with greater ease, flexibility, and decreased pain. Improvement in abdominal and back strength are thought to result from the combination of release techniques and exercises. The difficulty in resolving some of the areas is hypothesized to be due to the chronic positioning of these muscles by the spinal curve.

This case report demonstrates improvements in a patient's function following treatment that includes Positional Release. These improvements, in part, are due to the patient becoming more aware of her curve and the effects it has on her muscular function and dysfunction. She tends to substitute with muscles that are overworked and eventually became stuck in patterns, due to the inability of other muscles to assist in her everyday functions. The release techniques may have helped retrain her muscles or put them at a better mechanical advantage to work.

Idiopathic scoliosis is the most common type of lateral curvature of the spine, accounting for 65% of structural scoliosis found in adolescent patients.[2] One obstacle to the resolution of idiopathic scoliosis is the lack of an identifiable factor as the sole cause.[3] Although a cause for the patient's scoliosis is not identified, some success was achieved in treating the dysfunction apparently related to the scoliosis. Continued research is needed to determine the best treatment for individuals with adolescent idiopathic scoliosis. In addition, the focus should also include treatment of the psychological effects of this disorder.

Perhaps, too, as proficiency is improved with these techniques, more consistent results will be obtained. The tender areas diminished in number, but at times, their locations were puzzling (right versus left) and the patient's response to the treatment varied.

This therapist shows a great deal of insight regarding patient care and treatment potentiality, as shown by her lengthy discussion of the case. Many of her observations illuminate important points made in this publication. She shows a very good understanding of the connection between the patient's athletic activities and their impact on treatment results. In fact, she confirmed a specific overuse through palpation.

The fact that the symptoms were variable and changeable has a lot to do with the patient's continued athletic activities and the complex nature of the patient's dysfunction. Idopathic scoliosis is most likely unique to each individual's chronic use and holding patterns. This therapist was able to correlate muscular patterns of tightness with specific activity, which shows a high level of expertise required in these cases.

The mention of awareness as part of the Positional Release treatment benefits is also accurate and appropriate. It is interesting that, without any known restrictions given by the therapist, the patient decided to temporarily stop her athletic activities and give herself rest and recovery time. This most likely is also due to increased awareness on the patient's part and may be very beneficial during a time of such profound structural and functional change.

References

1. Keim H. *The Adolescent Spine.* New York: Grune and Stratton; 1976:6.
2. Cassella M, Hall J. Current treatment approaches in the nonoperative and operative management of adolescent idopathic scoliosis. *Physical Therapy.* 1991;71:897.
3. Kain J, Weiselfish S. Integrated manual therapy protocol for treatment of idiopathic scoliosis: A new concept. *Advances in Physical Therapy.* 1992;3:8–9.

21

Case Study 4. Myofascial Pain Syndrome

Heidi E. Baumeister, P.T., MHS program, University of Indianapolis
Edited comments by instructor Denise Deig, M.S.P.T., appear within rules.

Patient History

The patient is a 47-year-old woman with chronic neck and scapular pain, which began in January 1994. The patient reports moving and lifting many heavy boxes at the time of onset, with a gradual increase in neck and left scapular pain over the next few weeks. She was referred for physical therapy at that time and treated with ultrasound, electrical stimulation, moist heat, and a light exercise program. The patient reported improvement at the time of discharge from therapy, except she was unable to return to her normal lifting activities due to pain in the left arm.

The pain continued to improve gradually with occasional minor irritation reported until October 1997. At that time, she reported a gradual onset of left inferior and lateral breast pain that progressed to her left neck, shoulder, and scapular region. Gynecological work up, including multiple mammograms, found no abnormality. In June 1998, she was referred to a physiatrist for neck and shoulder pain, as her breast pain had decreased at the time. She was diagnosed with myofacial pain syndrome and referred to physical therapy. Her past medical history is otherwise unremarkable.

The patient is employed as a legal secretary for a large law firm and reports stress at work due to understaffing. She is married and has a teenage daughter.

Subjective Information

The patient reports moderate pain throughout the day that increases with work activities by evening. Upon evaluation she reports pain is 6/10 (with 10 being most severe). Ibuprofen and massage help to decrease her pain. Patient reports occasional numbness in her left upper extremity. She denies any difficulty sleeping or headaches. Coughing and swallowing do not increase pain. She reports that pain is constant at work and makes work difficult but does not limit function. Her goal is to decrease pain at work.

Objective Findings

Patient has a forward head posture, rounded shoulders, and bilaterally protracted scapulae. Active range of motion (AROM) of the cervical spine: flexion = 80°, extension = 45°, right rotation = 60° with pain, left rotation = 70°, side-bending right and left = 30° with pain on left side-bending. AROM of upper extremities is within normal limits (WNLs).

Cervical manual muscle tests (MMTs) is WNLs except as follows: flexion and left rotation = 4. Upper extremity MMTs is WNLs except as follows: left shoulder flexion = 4+, left external rotation = 4 (right = 4+), left internal rotation = 4+, left biceps = 4+ with pain, left triceps = 4 (right = 4+).

Deep tendon reflexes of biceps and triceps WNLs. Sensation is intact in cervical spine and both upper extremities. Vertebral artery test is negative. Drop arm test, Speed's test, and supraspinatus test are all negative with inconsistent pain reported in the left neck and shoulder girdle. Upper limb tension test is positive for medial arm pain with wrist and elbow extension and shoulder in 90° abduction. Special tests are performed according to Magee's *Orthopedic Physical Assessment*.[1]

Palpation reveals point tenderness, muscle tightness, and decreased tissue mobility in left cervical paraspinals, upper trapezius, scalenes, and rhomboids. Trigger points are noted lateral to C_6, in the upper trapezius near the levator scapula insertion, along the medial border of scapulae, and in the teres major muscle. Right neck and shoulder girdle muscles are negative to palpation.

Treatment Goals

1. Decrease muscle tissue tightness and trigger points.
2. Increase postural awareness.
3. Increase strength of left upper extremity and postural muscles.
4. Decrease pain with AROM of cervical spine.
5. Decrease pain with work activities.

Treatment

To determine the appropriate Positional Release technique, the patient was reassessed for point tenderness during each treatment. All release techniques were performed one to three times, until a significant decrease in tenderness was palpated.

Treatment 1

The patient is evaluated and instructed in using a proper ergonomic setup at her workstation to reduce stress on the neck and shoulders. The patient is given written instructions. Ultrasound is performed to the left upper trapezius and posterior shoulder region at 1.5 w/cm^2 for 5 minutes.

Treatment 2

The patient is instructed and monitored performing upper trapezius stretching and strengthening of scapular retractors using theraband, with written instructions given. Positional Release techniques are performed to the left lower trapezius and rhomboids. Ultrasound is performed as before.

Treatment 3

Chin tucks, scapular retractions, and shoulder circles are added to the home exercise program. Other exercises are reviewed and performed. Positional Release is done to the left levator scapulae, rhomboids, and upper trapezius muscles. Ultrasound is performed as before.

Treatment 4

The home exercise program is reviewed and an upper body bike and corner stretch added. Positional Release is done to the lower trapezius, levator scapula, and rhomboids. Ultrasound is performed, as before, followed by moist heat as patient complains of increased soreness today. Patient reports increased stress at work.

Treatment 5

The home exercise program is reviewed. Positional Release is given only to rhomboids, followed by ultrasound, as before.

Patient Response

After each treatment, point tenderness is reassessed, and the patient gives a subjective report of her response. At the end of each treatment, point tenderness is eliminated or reduced. The patient reports decreased pain after each treatment. If the patient is not working the day of her treatment, she reports the pain relief lasts through the next day. Generally, the patient reports some level of pain would return when she works following her treatment but not to the previous level.

The patient's postural awareness increased as did pain-free cervical-spine AROM. She continues to complain of left shoulder and upper trapezius pain, with a 50% improvement since her initial visit. Her physical therapy continues, with a decrease in the use of ultrasound and continued Positional Release and strengthening treatment. The therapist estimates that she will be seen for four to six additional visits, decreasing frequency to one time a week.

Discussion

Although the trigger points on the patient were not measured, using pressure dolorimetry, substantial relief of tenderness (50% decrease) is reported by the patient. Also, the gradual improvement in pain reported indicates there is some amount of carryover from treatment to treatment. It is important to note that Positional Release is not the entire treatment as it is used in combination with other treatments. Encouragement of stress management and modification of activities is also important in reducing and maintaining the patient's pain level. Through Positional Release, trigger point activity can be reduced, which results in decreased pain with functional activities.

This case study shows a good understanding and application of Positional Release as presented. The therapist reassesses with each visit and modifies her treatment program according to her findings. She also does a great job of integrating Positional Release and other treatment methods, including use of modalities, exercise, and postural retraining. This therapist shows a good awareness of the role the patient's stress and other work-related activities play in treatment and response. A 50% reduction in symptoms is a good response for five treatments of such a chronic condition.

Reference

1. Magee DJ. *Orthopedic Physical Assessment*. Philadelphia: W.B. Saunders Co.; 1992:117–121.

22

Case Study 5. Low Back Pain

Stacey M. Reeves, P.T., MHS Program, University of Indianapolis
Edited comments by instructor Denise Deig, M.S.P.T., appear within rules.

Patient History

The patient is a 50-year-old woman who sustained a back injury on June 2, while moving a hospital bed when trying to set up a patient for an EEG. She reports that she was quickly reaching down for the brake of the bed, while moving and pushing the bed, as the mechanism of injury. She reports an immediate "grab" in her low back, which worsened as the day progressed. The patient reports that she continues to work after the injury with limitations regarding moving beds, patients, and transfers, which require assistance. The patient was referred to outpatient physical therapy on June 16, with orders to evaluate and treat her low back pain three times a week for three weeks. She had a magnetic resonance imaging (MRI) the previous week but the results are not known to date.

Past medical history includes high blood pressure, thyroid disease, gallbladder surgery, and a hysterectomy. The patient has a history of a previous back injury in 1988, when she fell on a wet surface at work. With this previous injury, she was unable to work for two years and in physical therapy for 18 months. She reports that she has managed well since her return to work in 1990. She states that, since the initial injury, she has had some type of back pain continuously, although it is manageable.

Subjective Information

The patient's chief complaint is lower back pain with some radiation into the left buttocks to the hip. The pain is described as "grabbing." Sitting or a "wrong move" makes the pain worse, while lying down makes the pain better. She reports that the pain has improved 50% from this recent onset with home treatment of ice, heat, transcutaneous electrical nerve stimulation (TENS), stretching, and Advil. The pain ranges 6–10/10 (with 10 being most severe pain) and is constant. She reports numbness and tingling in the right upper-lateral thigh, which has been present since her 1988 injury, with no change from recent injury. Functionally, she reports that pain is her primary limiting factor. She states, "I have to stop when it gets to hurting too bad." Her goal from physical therapy is to "get relief from the grabbing pain and be able to stand and work for a longer period."

Objective Findings

The lumbar spine range of motion (ROM) is limited, with 50% forward flexion and 10° extension with pain. Other lumbar and cervical spine and extremity motions are within normal limits. Strength is normal except for bilateral hip flexors (right = 4–, left = 3+), knee flexors and extensors (right = 4+, left = 4–), and extensor hallicus longus (right and left = 4).

The patient presents increased sympathetic activity, as demonstrated by upper respiratory breathing and increased muscle tone of bilateral hip adductors and internal rotators. Trigger points are noted in the bilateral iliopsoas, right quadratus lumborum, and anterior T_{12} tenderpoint (Strain-CounterStrain®)[1] on the left ilium. Muscle spasm and guarding are noted throughout the lumbar area bilaterally with a decrease in all spinal curves.

The patient presents an overall decrease in her functional ability and mobility due to the increased pain, increased adverse neural tension, decreased range of motion, decreased strength, increased muscle spasm and tone, and increased point tenderness in muscles noted above. She requires minimal assistance for moving from a supine to a sitting position due to pain but can move from a sitting to a supine position independently, although slowly and painfully. Trunk movement is guarded during transitional movements and her gait pattern is slow and cautious.

Treatment Goals

1. Decrease "grabbing" pain during bending and with standing.
2. Independence in a home exercise program.
3. Return the patient to her previous activity level and functional abilities at home and work with little or no pain.

Treatment and Patient Response

Treatment 1

Evaluation is carried out. Positional Release is given to bilateral iliopsoas, with immediate pain reduction reported. The patient is instructed in Feldenkrais® rotating and warming exercises and diaphragmatic breathing.

Treatment 2

The patient reports significant pain relief after the first session. The MRI results show no abnormalities. Positional Release is given for bilateral iliopsoas, diaphragm, right quadratus, and left anterior T_{12} tenderpoint with Strain-CounterStrain. Point tenderness and pain decrease following the session, and the patient reports a "warming" sensation in the low back. The patient is instructed in self-release of bilateral iliospsoas for a home program.

Treatment 3

The patient reports a decrease in low back pain and numbness in the right thigh. She is better able to handle work stress with the decreased pain intensity. Pain is 4/10 prior to treatment and 2/10 posttreatment. Point tenderness is decreased but still noted. The treatment given is as in session 2. She reports the "deep ache" and "grabbing" pain in her back are gone after treatment.

Treatment 4

The patient reports that back pain has returned to the level it was before the recent injury, ranked 2/10. The treatment given is as before, with sacrum Positional Release techniques added. Her gait is observed to be normal and transitional movements are done with more ease, although moving from a supine to a sitting position remains slow. The patient is using a TENS unit at home regularly.

Treatment 5

The patient has seen her doctor and has been released from his care. He wants her to finish her last week of therapy as per original orders. She reports an increase in pain with increased work stress. She now is aware of a change from diaphragmatic to upper chest breathing with stress. The patient is given handouts to instruct family members in performing Positional Releases on iliopsoas, quadratus lumborum, and Strain-CounterStrain on anterior T_{12}. Recommendations are given for a walking program to improve cardiovascular fitness and help with stress reduction. The treatment was done as previously. Due to the patient's progress level, the therapist did not recommend finishing her last two visits. However, the patient wanted to continue, due to increased work stress and a need for further education regarding breathing patterns.

Treatments 6 and 7

The patient does not show up for these appointments and cancels her remaining two appointments. When contacted by phone, she reports to the therapist that she has returned to her previous functional level with a significant decrease in pain, and therefore need not continue with therapy. She is walking 15 minutes a day and will progress as able. Her husband is doing Positional Releases on her as needed. She feels her goals with physical therapy have been met and she is better able to deal with stress at work with no increase in back pain.

Discussion

The patient was seen a total of five treatment sessions. She met her goals with a full return to previous functional level with little to no pain. With the assistance of her family, she is independent in her home program.

I feel this is an excellent patient on which to perform Positional Release. She gives excellent feedback on what does or does not feel good. She has a lot of knowledge regarding exercise, self-care, and pain management due to her previous injury. She does a wonderful job learning diaphragmatic breathing, especially in stressful situations.

The nature of her injury, in which she made a quick and jerky movement while moving a bed, fits with the "panic response" of a neuromuscular dysfunction. The overall hyperactivity of her sympathetic system also fits with the concept of the "facilitated segment."

This patient seems very "high strung," and I anticipated a psychological issue in discharging her. She did not seem to want to "let go." Therefore, I was shocked when she canceled her last two appointments due to feeling much better. I also was very pleased with the wonderful, immediate effects Positional Release had on her as well as some of my other patients. I feel as though I gained a special "tool" to help educate others.

This therapist also shows an excellent grasp of the concepts presented in this book. She identifies a clear mechanism of injury and treats the involved anterior structures that one would think to be in dysfunction from the history given. This most likely speeded the healing process, as indicated by the drastic and rapid decrease in pain. I find it interesting that the right thigh numbness from an 11-year-old injury also resolved to some extent by the third treatment of the current injury.

The therapist has a good grasp of this patient's stress and psychological factors and their impact on treatment. This aspect was treated appropriately with a diaphragmatic breathing emphasis, although this patient may be a candidate for further stress management intervention.

To a great extent, this patient already was schooled in the use of exercise, TENS, ice, and heat for self-care and a home program. She most likely would have benefited minimally if at all to a physical therapy approach providing only more of the same. The recently acquired Positional Release skills allowed this therapist to provide considerable relief from suffering and restoration of function in this patient in a short amount of time.

Reference

1. Jones LH, with Kusunose RS, Goering EK. *Jones Strain-CounterStrain*. Boise, ID: Jones Strain-CounterStrain; 1995.

23

Case Study 6. Total Knee Replacement

Andrea Phillips, P.T., MHS Program, University of Indianapolis
Edited comments by instructor Denise Deig, M.S.P.T., appear within rules.

Patient History and Subjective Findings

The patient is a 74-year-old woman who had her first total (left) knee replacement (TKR) done in 1976 secondary to degenerative joint disease. Her knee was manipulated four times (while the patient was under anesthesia) within the same year due to poor range of motion. The patient attained 0–85° of knee range of motion (ROM) and functional independence.

In 1998, the patient started having knee pain and instability requiring her to wear a knee immobilizer. She also required a straight cane for ambulation due to pain. Radiological findings showed a loosening of the prosthesis. The patient had a preoperative evaluation done on June 6, 1999, and surgery (second TKR) was done three days later with no complications.

The patient was seen for home physical therapy two weeks later, after discharge from a subacute treatment facility. The patient's primary complaint was restricted motion and pain with movement and weight bearing activities. Pain was rated 6/10 (with 10 being the most severe pain). Pain was reported to be in the left anterior-lateral aspect of quadriceps with radiation to patella.

Objective Findings

1. Left knee active range of motion (AROM) 10–70° with an empty end feel.
2. Grade 1 edema in knee joint and leg.
3. Strength within normal limits except for left leg, 4/5 for hamstrings and iliopsoas and 3/5 for quadriceps.
4. Gait pattern with antalgic limp.
5. Ambulation over level and uneven surfaces with use of walker.
6. Patient requires assistance with step climbing.

Treatment Goals

1. Increase ROM in the left knee.
2. Decrease pain.
3. Improve function for sitting in a car and gait.
4. Ambulate with straight cane as before.
5. Return to previous level of function and activity.

Treatment and Patient Response

Treatment 1

Initial evaluation and treatment given with a home program of short and long arch quadriceps strengthening, ankle pumps, and knee flexion and extension, followed by ice. Gait training is with a large-base quad cane on level and uneven surfaces and up and down three steps. Weight-bearing exercises, such as single leg stance, also are performed.

Upon the initial evaluation, this therapist has not yet taken the Positional Release course and, therefore, no releases are given in the first treatment session.

Treatment 2

Positional Release is given to left quadriceps while patient is supine. Pretreatment pain was 6/10, post treatment pain is 1/10 with report of numbness over the previously painful area (anterior-lateral quadriceps). The ROM increased from 0–85° to 0–93°, with less pain after the releases.

Treatment 3

The patient reports no return of pain, no numbness, and increased ease of movement, especially freedom with knee bending. Positional Release is given to the hamstrings and quadriceps, followed by isometrics. The AROM improved from 0–95° prior to treatment to 0–100° post-treatment. Patient is ambulating independently, with a large-based quad cane, with no antalgic gait.

Further Treatment

Treatment now focuses on gait training with a straight cane and stair climbing. Patient had an 18-inch-high step, which required standby assistance for safety.

It is unclear, from this case study, how many additional visits this patient received before discharge.

Discussion

Positional Release to the quadriceps is used to decrease pain and facilitate relaxation in this patient. The patient reports immediate relief with the release done only one time. The patient complained of this pain since surgery, so this treatment intervention is successful. Quadricep and hamstring releases are done to clear out any tension in the joint and allow the muscles to function more normally, resulting in increased ROM. Isometrics are done to assist with increasing muscle strength in both hamstrings and quadriceps.

The patient complained of pain over the anterior-lateral aspect of the left leg distal to the patella with radiation down to the ankle. She reported that it felt like she was "kicked in the shin by a horse." Positional Release to the anterior tibialis, which was the only muscle that could have been involved, is unsuccessful. Soft tissue mobilization is also attempted without success. The patient was referred back to the physician. A circulatory work up and X rays found no abnormalities. At the time of discharge, the patient still complains of pain but to a lesser extent.

Positional Release is very useful with this patient and assists in achieving the goals of increasing ROM, decreasing pain, and improving strength. A few limitations are noted in implementing this technique. The prone position for the hamstring release is not very comfortable for this patient and so it is difficult for the patient to relax. She cannot tolerate the supine position with the leg over the edge of the bed either, because it increases stretching of the quadriceps and pain. Also, this patient has tenderness over the painful area on the left leg. This makes it difficult to palpate and feel for any softening of tissues, since just touching her increases her pain.

I include this case study, in part, to observe a successful application in a home care setting. The therapist's struggle with placing the patient in a hamstring release position is of interest, because it highlights the need to accommodate the releases to the circumstances at hand. I am unclear as to how the therapist released the hamstrings, but I would suggest a semi-prone or side-lying position, using pillows for support, with the involved leg up. The supine "leg off the table" hamstring release most likely would be too extreme, since probably there is primary quadricep involvement due to the surgical and manipulative history and patient's dramatic response to the initial quadricep release. It also would be difficult to obtain a less extreme position in the home without the availability of a high-low table.

The left lower leg pain also is of interest in this case. I would not agree that the anterior tibialis is the only structure that could be responsible for the pain. I am curious about the relationship to the primary complaint of left anterior-lateral pain from quadriceps to patella. The pain that extends from the patella to the ankle may have been part of a larger fascial strain pattern related to previous knee joint disease, surgery, or trauma from four surgical manipulations. I would have continued to treat and explore the possibilities of joint restrictions coming from the ankle or knee or other possible referred pain from a posterior calf, ankle, or foot muscle. If the therapist was able to find the exact source of the problem, it may have cleared as easily as the quadriceps pain did in this case.

24

Case Study 7. Cervical Whiplash Injury

Lynne Patterson, P.T., MHS Program, University of Indianapolis
Edited comments by instructor Denise Deig, M.S.P.T., appear within rules.

Patient History and Subjective Information

The patient is a 30-year-old woman, who works as a secretary. She was referred to physical therapy by her family physician after sustaining injuries to her neck approximately two weeks previously as a result of a motor vehicle accident (MVA). The patient recalls injury of a hyperflexion-hyperextension type. She has been on Motrin and off work since the MVA.

The patient's chief complaint is of "sharp, burning, and stabbing right-sided neck pain that feels like a hot poker." Symptoms increase with sustained positions, driving, and turning to the left. The patient also reports frequent headaches and denies any radicular symptoms. She reports no significant past medical history. X rays show no abnormalities.

Objective Findings

The patient presents a poor sitting posture, forward head, rounded shoulders, and a decreased lumbar lordosis. Active range of motion (AROM) of the cervical spine reveals a 25% decrease in left rotation and side-bending, with the complaint of right cervical pain. Passive ROM reveals pain at the end range of left rotation and side-bending greater than right. Significant pain is noted with resisted right-side bending and flexion.

A neurological screen found no abnormalities. All other special tests also found no cause for the pain. Palpation reveals two significant trigger points in right distal sternocleidomastoid with spasm. The C_4 through C_6 vertebrae are flexed, side-bent, and rotated to the right. Mild point tenderness anterior to the C_4–C_6 transverse processes on the right also is noted.

Treatment Goals

1. Increase pain-free cervical range of motion.
2. Decrease cervical asymmetry.
3. Improve posture.
4. Increase pain-free cervical strength.
5. Return patient to previous level of function. Patient's goals were to return to work, bike riding, and aerobics.

Treatment and Patient Response

Treatments 1–5

Initial treatments consist of ultrasound to right sternocleidomastoid (SCM) followed by stretching, using contract-relax methods. Muscle energy techniques are used to increase extension, side-bending, and rotation to left at C_4–C_5. Ice is given after these techniques.

The patient is instructed in proper postural mechanics and ice for a home program. No significant decrease in right SCM tenderness or any decrease in cervical asymmetry is noted in the initial treatment protocol.

Treatments 1–5 are given prior to the Positional Release course, and treatments 6–13 are given after taking the weekend course.

Treatment 6

Moist heat is given to the cervical region, followed by Positional Release to the right SCM. The position of release is found to be in almost full flexion with right side-bending and slight left rotation. Release is held for 60 seconds and repeated twice, with no "release" palpated by the therapist. Point tenderness continues as before.

Treatment 7

The patient returns with the same complaints and a slight decrease in intensity of sharp pain. Positional Release is given to the right SCM following moist heat, as before. Minimal release is palpated and mild tenderness prevails at the end of the session, although decreased from the start. Patient receives ice in the release position following the releases.

Treatment 8

The patient reports no carryover of decreased point tenderness from the last treatment and symptoms are unchanged. A reevaluation is due and carried out. A significant right levator scapulae trigger point is noted and released with the patient supine, with a 75-second hold. The right SCM then is released. After 30 seconds, the patient begins to cry. After the cervical spine is slowly returned to neutral, the patient is given a drink of water. She is questioned as to why the sudden outburst, to which she answered, "I don't know, I just felt like crying." The patient and therapist are allowed to rest for 10 minutes. On return, palpation of the right SCM reveals a significant decrease in spasm and minimal tenderness. Ice is given to the SCM in a shortened position.

Treatment 9

The patient reports being almost free of symptoms, with only "intermittent twinges of right-side pain." No tenderness is found in the right levator scapula. The right SCM is released twice after finding the most distal point tender. Isometrics into extension and left side-bending are given at various angles until the cervical spine is almost neutral. No point tenderness is noted on palpation. The right SCM again is iced in the shortened position. The patient is instructed in self-release for the SCM and told to continue ice with the home program.

Treatment 10

The patient reports doing well. She has returned to work and reports compliance with the home program. She complains of intermittent upper trapezius "soreness." No point tenderness is palpated. The SCM is released, followed by isometrics and ice, as before.

Treatment 11

The patient continues to do well. The treatment is repeated as in session 10.

Treatment 12

Reevaluation reveals full pain-free cervical ROM and strength. No cervical asymmetry or tenderness is noted. She is treated as before, with Positional Release, isometrics, and ice. Instruction for home program and postural reeducation was reviewed.

Treatment 13

The patient returns one week later with no complaints, except for intermittent upper trapezius soreness, which she relates to stress. She has returned to some light aerobic activity, with minimal complaints of lower extremity soreness. The patient is instructed to continue the home program for one month. She is to call the clinic if any of her previous symptoms return. To date, the therapist has not heard from this patient.

Discussion

Unfortunately, the therapist does not include a discussion section in her case report. I would have been interested in her response and feelings regarding the emotional release this patient had during treatment. The emotional release is triggered by release of the most involved musculature, the SCM, but not until after the levator scapular trigger is located and treated. This is an interesting example of the importance of treatment sequencing. The therapist's response to the patient's crying is appropriate in offering water and rest to give her time to integrate the release. I would like to note how little response there is to the indirect or other procedures prior to the emotional release and how little treatment is really required after this session. She includes the following reflection in her introduction.

Although manual therapy may seem to be a dying art in some realms, as technological advances make us more dependent on machines than our hands, some techniques continue to smolder and refuse to die out. Frequently, new light may be shed on some old approaches, while other techniques may be introduced. This is a case study of a relatively new technique called *Positional Release*.

25

Case Study 8. Degenerative Disc Disease of Lumbar Spine with Radiculopathy

Denise Deig, M.S.P.T., G.C.F.P.

Patient History

This 29-year-old male firefighter presented with a history of chronic low-back pain, which originated in 1989 or 1990. In 1993, the back pain became more significant, with episodes of debilitating pain lasting two or three days. Pain was localized in the right side of the back and radiated down the right leg. He reported several work-related incidents that had contributed to his condition; however, this patient was not receiving workers compensation. In particular, he related a significant back injury, which occurred in July 1995, that involved lifting a heavy person while twisting. He reported that, since this incident, his pain and symptoms have progressively worsened. By Fall 1996, he had to quit working out on a regular basis due to the back condition, in part because of an additional injury he had sustained while lifting weights. The patient wrote, "At this time, 25% of my life was spent experiencing some type of back pain. Something as simple as waking up in the morning at work would set it off, and I could only (at best) walk crouched over for several days to two weeks."

In February 1999, he had an MRI, which showed three compressed discs in the lumbar spine, and he was diagnosed with advanced degenerative disc disease for his age. He was given exercises by the neurologist at that time but reported that, "either my back hurt too bad to do them consistently or the exercises seemed to excite my weak back condition."

The patient reported a recent exacerbation of his back condition, which occurred on December 14, 1999, that involved normal work-related activities but no actual injury or incident he could recall. He summarized his condition with, "I've had growing back pain in the last year and a half. Life can be broken down into thirds; a third in some pain, a third in real pain, and the last part relatively normal."

Subjective Information

The patient reported low-back pain with radicular pain in a posterior distribution in both lower extremities, which alternated between left and right legs. The right lower-extremity radicular pain went to the calf, while the left lower-extremity radicular pain went to the foot. He also reported some pelvic floor symptomology, with increased pain with bowel movements and urination and testicular pain when the back pain was most severe. Pain was rated as ranging from 2–10, with 10 being the most severe pain.

This patient was unable to work out or lift weights, as too much activity or exercise significantly aggravated his symptoms. He had run several marathons in the past and worked out on a regular basis until his back condition limited his functional abilities. The patient was concerned about his ability to continue working as a firefighter, due to the progressive nature of his back condition. He had a second job, as owner of a lawn care service, which also required intense physical activity.

Previously, the patient had been seen at a hospital-based sports medicine clinic for two or three physical therapy visits in 1996. He received primarily theraband exercises, which were of no significant help to him.

Objective Findings

On initial evaluation on January 3, 2000, his range of motion (ROM) was limited in the lumbar spine with 50° flexion and 5° extension with pain. Hamstring tightness was noted bilaterally, left more than right, with 40° on left and 55° on right with straight leg raise. Driving tolerance was 5 minutes and sitting tolerance was 15 minutes.

Movement of the lumbar and lower thoracic spine were extremely guarded in all activities and movement observed. The patient was in a forward flexed posture with an inability to stand fully erect. A slight right lateral shift of the trunk on the pelvis also was noted. Poor sitting and standing posture were noted, especially due to forward flexion of spine.

Structural dysfunction was noted with a positive standing flexion test on the right and a right anterior ilium rotation. Severe lumbosacral compression was present. Palpation revealed severe hypertonus in the right thoracic and lumbar paraspinals, right quadratus lumborum, left piriformis, and bilateral iliopsoas muscles.

Treatment Goals

1. Increase ROM in the lumbar spine 10–15° by the end of one month.
2. Decrease pain rating to 2–6/10 by the end of one month.
3. Resolve soft tissue and joint dysfunction throughout the pelvis, spine, and lower extremities by discharge.
4. Decrease lower extremity radicular pain by discharge.
5. Independence in self-care and home exercise by discharge.
6. Return patient to his previous level of activity with regard to exercise and work by discharge.

Treatment

Treatment 1

Physical therapy evaluation plus 15 minutes each of manual therapy and neuromuscular reeducation are carried out. Treatment includes Positional Release muscular application for bilateral iliopsoas, left piriformis, right quadratus lumborum, lumbar and thoracic paraspinals (right more than left). Right anterior ilium rotation and right lateral shift are addressed with Positional Release joint application followed by isometrics. Lumbosacral decompression is given with Positional Release followed by a direct technique. Movement work is given for the pelvis, spine, and lower extremities from a flexed, supine position.

Treatment 2

One week later, the patient returns for therapy and reports some relief following the first session, with a decrease in left lower extremity radicular pain. He reports that taking muscle relaxants prior to bedtime also seems beneficial in decreasing symptoms. His posture is noted to be improved, with less forward flexion. The treatment includes neuromuscular reeducation for one hour. Positional Release is given with the release of neuromuscular dysfunction to the bilateral iliopsoas, diaphragm, abdominals, and left piriformis muscles as well as joint releases to lumbar spine and sacrum (general release, left sacrotuberous and bilateral posterior sacroiliac ligaments). Movement work is given to bilateral lower extremities (on the left more than the right), pelvis, and spine.

Treatment 3

Two days later, the patient again is seen for treatment. At that time, he notes significant improvement, with decreased low-back pain and decreased left lower-extremity radicular pain. He reports a new awareness of pain in the left proximal tibia-fibular region in the lateral aspect. The treatment includes neuromuscular reeducation for 45 minutes and therapeutic exercise for 15 minutes. Neuromuscular dysfunctions are addressed with Positional Release to left iliopsoas muscle and joint releases to the left tibia-fibula (proximal more that distal), left hip, lumbar spine, and sacrum, as before. Movement work is given to both lower extremities, pelvis, and spine. The patient is given a home exercise program with diaphragmatic breathing and bilateral knee to chest movement explorations, with circles and figure eights progressing to random movement activities. Patient is doing so well that the next several appointments are canceled. He is scheduled to be reevaluated in one month.

Patient Response

The patient is not seen at the scheduled appointment time, due to the therapist being ill. He is contacted by phone approximately two and a half months after the last visit to determine if he should be scheduled for further treatment or be discharged.

The patient reports that he is doing very well and therefore needed no further treatment. He reports pain only with extreme activity. When it does occur, it is present in the left buttocks and low back and is reported to range from 1–2/10. Mild tightness is noted in the lower back with some motions.

The posture of the patient is improved in both sitting and standing. He reports no limitations to driving or sitting activities. He has returned to working full time at both jobs, as a firefighter and in his lawn care business. He has returned to his previous level of activity with weight lifting, stretching, and strengthening exercises, although these are intentionally less strenuous than before. The patient reports that the difference before and after physical therapy treatment is like "night and day."

Discussion

This patient responded extremely well to Positional Release techniques and Feldenkrais®-type movement reeducation. I anticipated that he would require a much longer period of care due to the chronic nature of his problem and the physical demands of his daily life.

The patient had very obvious structural dysfunction of his pelvis, spine, and left lower extremity that was responsive to indirect work. The neuromuscular dysfunction and hypertonicity of the involved muscles kept this patient locked in a chronic holding pattern and a state of facilitation so severe that simple movement and activities of daily living exacerbated it. The iliopsoas, diaphragm, and abdominal muscles contributed significantly to the forward flexed posture and probably were part of the original mechanism of injury, although this is unclear from the complicated past history with multiple insults. Patient had secondary joint restrictions in the left lower extremity, which became more evident as his primary pelvic and lumbar spine restrictions began to clear.

This case study is an excellent example of how appropriate physical therapy treatment with a primary focus on Positional Release technique can assist a patient in returning to a very high functional status. Exercise was an inappropriate intervention for this patient, who was in a chronic state of facilitation, until the underlying soft tissue and joint dysfunctions were treated successfully and resolved. All goals were either met or exceeded in a shorter time period than expected, possibly due in part to the patient's age and general condition. Nearly 100% return of function in three visits for someone with a chronic, 10-year-old condition is a very effective outcome, worthy of further investigation.

Index

Page references with "t" denote tables; "f" denote figures.